Yoga Self-Taught provides a complete handbook for anyone who wants to learn yoga. If you cannot attend yoga classes, or want to supplement what you have learnt at them or simply prefer to teach yourself at home, then *Yoga Self-Taught* is the ideal book for you.

It describes over 200 exercises and positions for beginners in the fullest possible detail with the help of over 100 photographs and numerous illustrations, showing both the *right* way and the *wrong* way to perform them. The full yoga breathing system is described in detail – and for every exercise included, the benefits and effects are clearly described. *Yoga Self-Taught* provides a simple but very effective method of relaxation.

Twenty-five years' practice and nearly fifteen years' teaching at the Integral Yoga Institute in Brussels have made André van Lysebeth one of Europe's most experienced teachers. Founder and President of the Belgian Yoga Federation, he has taught students from all over the world.

'In a class of its own.'   *Healthy Living*

D1051101

Yoga Self-Taught

ANDRÉ VAN LYSEBETH

London
UNWIN PAPERBACKS
Boston   Sydney

First published in Great Britain by
George Allen & Unwin 1971
Reprinted 1974
First published in Unwin Paperbacks 1978
Reprinted 1980
Reprinted 1983
Reprinted 1985

UNWIN® PAPERBACKS
40 Museum Street, London WC1A 1LU, UK

Unwin Paperbacks
Park Lane, Hemel Hempstead, Herts HP2 4TE

George Allen & Unwin Australia Pty Ltd,
8 Napier Street, North Sydney, NSW 2060, Australia

Translated from *J'Apprends le Yoga* (*Flammarion*) by Carola
Congreve
Copyright © André van Lysebeth 1968
This translation copyright © George Allen & Unwin
(Publishers) Ltd 1971, 1978

British Library Cataloguing in Publication Data

Lysebeth, André van
  Yoga self-taught.
  1. Yoga, Hatha
  I. Title
  613.7   RA781.7   78-40453

  ISBN 0-04-149049-5

Printed and bound in Great Britain by
Hazell Watson & Viney Limited,
Member of the BPCC Group,
Aylesbury, Bucks

Foreword

Hatha-yoga is first and foremost a yoga – although this fact is often forgotten. The term 'yoga' which is in etymology related to the French 'joug' meaning 'yoke', a word reappearing in the adjective 'conjugal', is taken to have two principal meanings, which are furthermore closely connected. The state of yoga is that in which man is 'yoked together' with the Divine – an idea expressed in the word 're-ligion'. In a slightly different sense yoga signifies the state in which the 'apparent man' binds himself likewise to the 'real man' – that is to say, recovers his true nature and lives according to it. The *technique* of yoga is the discipline in whatever form it is practised, by which man attempts to attain the *state* of yoga.

According to the Hindu conception each and every technique, if followed assiduously and with concentration, can lead to the high level of consciousness which corresponds to the state of yoga. Thus it is possible to speak of the yoga of art, of science, grammar, of love, of the yoga of meditation, and so on. But this accepted, each yoga carries with it the practice of a severe and correct discipline.

There are traditionally four principal yogas to consider: the yoga of the exploration of the intellect to beyond the normal boundaries of the mind (Jnānayoga)[1]; the yoga of love centred on the Divine through an image of Itself or towards some object or person in whom the Divine is perceived (this is Bhakti-yoga); the yoga of inner concentration (Rāja-yoga), and the yoga of disinterested action undertaken more or less directly on behalf of the Divine (Karma-yoga)[2].

However complete in themselves each of these four yogas may be, it is not possible entirely to dissociate them one from another. The great sages have always laid stress on the one hand that, when one yoga is followed, it is usually at the very least dangerous to depart in any way whatever from its own set of fundamental rules, and on the other they have ruled that in the final analysis each yoga reunites one with the other. The pure Bhakti-yogi acquires automatically the supreme knowledge which is the goal of Jnāna-yoga; the

[1]See Swāmi Vivekānanda, *Jnâna-Yoga* (Paris, Albin Michel).
[2]See Swāmi Vivekānanda, *Les Yogas pratiques (Bhakti, Karma, Râja)* (Paris, Albin Michel).

pure jnāna-yogi culminates in the supreme love (para-bhakta), which the bhakti-yogi sets out to find[3]. Intensive practice in Rāja-yoga is almost indispensable in all the other yogas, and Karma-yoga can reach to such perfect completeness that Shrī Aurobindo, the greatest master of modern India, has seen in it the perfect yoga, that is to say the yoga which embraces all others[4].

In speaking of the practice of some specific yoga we do not seek to exclude the others, but we imply that the yoga in question supplies those who appeal to it, with a form of central ruling on which the others are hinged.

The outline becomes even less clear-cut, when it is seen that each yoga embodies in itself an endless number of variants, and that each master teaches a technique which he himself has devised; usually the one he has followed and into which he has consciously injected elements drawn from a variety of yogas.

Apart from these four great yogas and their diverse variants and combinations, other classic yogas exist, among them we should mention Mantra-yoga, Japayoga[5], Laya-yoga and the other tantric yogas, Agni-yoga, and Hatha-yoga, which is the one Westerners most often have in mind when they hear the word 'yoga'. All may be practised more or less in isolation—that is to say they may play a lesser or greater role in the composition of the individual yogas.

Although a true master or *guru* will never accept any candidate for teaching unless he considers objectively that his own brand of yoga is entirely suited to the would-be pupil, we should note that the greatest masters, those who have themselves attained the uttermost heights of spiritual development, see that every pupil throughout his training partakes of the particular discipline best suited to him[6].

This book deals with Hatha-yoga. At the outset, and a fairly long time ago, Hatha-yoga, seen merely as a complement of Rāja-yoga, was already an entity. While the great classicists of Hatha-dipika, Shiva Samhita, Goraksha Samhita, the most ancient of which date from the thirteenth century, are looked upon still largely as a tool in the practice of the other yogas, the yoga of the physical body

[3]See *L'Enseignement de Râmakrishna* (Paris, Albin Michel), 1167–99.
[4]See Shrī Aurobindo, *Le Guide du Yoga* (Paris, Albin Michel).
[5]See Swāmi Rāmdās, *Carnet de Pèlerinage* (Paris, Albin Michel).
[6]See Shrī Aurobindo, *Lettres* (Paris, Adyar), 3 Vols.

early assumed great importance. Although clearly within the framework of Hinduism, it has for a long time been practised in India by the adepts of other religions (Sikhs, Jains, Parsees, Mohammedans), sometimes under other names. Its goal is generally expressed by the term *nadi suddhi*, by which the yogis mean essentially the vitalization of the body, and the purification of the para-nervous system, which together constitute the *nadi*.

Hatha-yoga, at least as much as any of the other yogas, is open to a variety of uses and in itself contains a considerable number of variants. It is composed of two parts, the physical and the mental.

The physical part is composed essentially of two elements, the postures (asanas) and controlled respiration (prānayama). But it is the mental part which plays the determining role, and upon which depends to a great extent the effect derived from the physical practices: many Westerners make the greatest mistake in failing to afford it the importance it deserves.

Hatha-yoga practised in isolation, or as the main element in an individual composite yoga, can, according to the greatest of the Hindu specialists, suffice to guide the yogi to the highest degree of spiritual evolution. There have always been, and there are still in India today, the greatest sages who have never followed another discipline. They live, usually very withdrawn, often in the jungle or in the mountains, almost inaccessible to ordinary mortals, only rarely accepting pupils: those who in their view are capable of submitting themselves to unbelievably arduous practices, fraught with every sort of danger, danger into which it would be purest folly to stray without the guidance from day to day, if not from hour to hour, of a considerable master. This total Hatha-yoga, therefore is not for Westerners, and, what is more, the qualified teachers who represent it have never committed the fatal error of consigning its teachings to the written word, except into hermetically sealed and unusable texts. And this complete Hatha-yoga is normally –if not always–practised within the framework of the Hindu religion, that is to say its goal is the union or fusion with one of the gods of the Hindu Pantheon, or with Shiva or one of his Shaktis[7].

On the other hand, the first elements of Hatha-yoga, practised as a subordinate discipline are currently in use in India, not only by those who practise another yoga as their acknowledged discipline

[7]See Shankara, *Hymnes à Shiva* (Lyon, Derain).

to reach the higher levels of consciousness, but also by those who seek merely to harvest the physical and mental advantages without the anxiety involved in religious or spiritual development, general or specific.

It is these first principles which are practised by a growing number of Westerners today, either under the guidance of more or less experienced professors or through study based upon books illustrated with sketches or photographs. The benefit that can derive through the regular practice of the most elementary of the Hatha-yoga techniques is so greatly out of proportion to any effort demanded, that this yoga has spread through the West like wild-fire. Publications devoted to the subject are legion. The 'schools' allegedly teaching it are now innumerable. Many of them justify the gravest misgivings and the uninitiated who put themselves in such hands run a real risk. Even the easiest and seemingly least harmful of the exercises are not free from danger. But more disquieting still is that the encouraging results, obtainable in a relatively short time with a minimum of effort, may inspire the beginner to make light of the advice so constantly meted out to him to be careful and moderate, and he may throw himself hastily into dangerous techniques, leading to serious trouble in the respiratory, circulatory and nervous systems.

For over thirty years I have been trying to persuade the great Hindu masters to describe to Westerners – stressing any precautions necessary – exercises which may be undertaken with good results and in safety. Not one of these masters was sufficiently confident of the ability of Westerners, to comply with my request.

M. Van Lysebeth's book seems to come as near as any Westerner has so far, in bridging this gap. Wise enough to limit his aims to some very detailed description of a few of the main postures and the method of achieving them, he has done something of the utmost importance, which to my knowledge no Westerner has ever done before: he has made the most minute exposition of the physiological and other effects which the practice of the postures can bestow, the dangers to be avoided, any contra-indications and so on.

I believe this book to be entirely trustworthy, and I hope M. Van Lysebeth will complement it with other works, where he will describe, likewise in detail, and with the same warnings, a variety of other Hatha-yoga exercises.

JEAN HERBERT

Preface

The purpose of this book is to offer a study more detailed and accurate than any so far published. Hitherto (except for Iyengar's *Light on Yoga*) even the best works on the subject have confined themselves to the reproduction of photographs of the final posture, rarely showing intermediary stages. At the same time only the most fragmentary of instructions are given as to the technique of the postures, their variants, their duration, the order in which they should follow one another in a series of asanas, the method of breathing, how and where to concentrate the mind, the effects of the exercises and so on. The Westerner who has never lived in an ashram alongside the Master is forced to grope in the dark, and to consult the innumerable works on the subject (many of which have borrowed from each other!), in order to pick up scraps of knowledge, and so laboriously to piece together the correct technique.

One may indeed question the wisdom of indiscriminate publication, since for thousands of years yoga has been handed down in sworn secrecy by word of mouth from Master to disciple; and it might seem that the wish of the Masters, to reserve yoga to carefully selected adepts, should therefore be respected. We are sure that countless Westerners need yoga, especially Hatha-yoga, and that the number of adepts 'ripe' for mental and other forms of yoga is far greater than is generally believed. Why not, then, relay to them the invaluable techniques perfected by the Rishis? Even leaving out of account the fact that the harm–if harm it is–was done years ago! In yoga more than anywhere else, half-truths are disastrous–if one takes the responsibility for passing on knowledge, then at least one should offer complete instructions, rather than mere crumbs of information. Unless *every* detail necessary to the correct practice is given, then how much better to remain silent. Yet, as far as we know, no such exhaustive study has ever been attempted. A yogic asana is a technique of precision: the approximate has never had a place in yoga. One mistaken detail, apparently minuscule, may rob an exercise of an important part of its effect, and may even work counter to the end in view.

This study is interesting as much to those already practising yoga as to the beginner desirous of learning, but lacking the opportunity to take lessons. We shall therefore help you as reader to study one posture at a time. Before long you will possess a thorough knowledge of the exact technique of the great classics of yoga, and, from their practice, will harvest all the benefit and happiness which yoga well done can produce. Your daily session will become neither arduous nor routine, but will be the best moment of the day, impatiently awaited, or awaited with as much impatience as a would-be yogi ought properly to allow himself!

Each asana is made up of stages of ever-increasing difficulty: our study is based upon a medium stage which most Westerners can reach within a few weeks. Thanks to the precise nature of the instruction given here, beginners will be able to overcome the preliminary obstacles without any difficulty. For advanced pupils we shall, in each case, describe a more elaborate variant: in this way both kinds of reader will get something out of the book.

Contents

1. *Modern Man and Yoga*

What a time to be alive!

Never has mankind known such an evolutionary explosion. We have accomplished things beyond the wildest dreams of our ancestors. Our cosmonauts have eclipsed Icarus. Our scientists have penetrated to the heart of the atom, and from it have torn the most closely guarded secrets of nature: they have harnessed nuclear energy for domestic use. We lead a fairy-tale existence compared to that of former centuries. How sad we should take all this for granted!

We think nothing of sitting comfortably in an upholstered seat, flying over the Pole in our Boeing, while far below an atomic submarine cruises beneath the ice-cap. And in our aeroplanes we . . . sleep.

No need to go back as far as the Romans: it is enough to imagine the astonishment of Louis XIV or Queen Anne faced with television or an ordinary tape-recorder.

Like spoilt children we complain if the transmission from Telstar is a little blurred. The motor-car is such an everyday affair that we think nothing of driving down the motorway at 70 m.p.h.

We dial a number and at the other end of the wire hundreds, even thousands of miles away, a well-loved voice replies. Loved, that is providing it is not the Inspector of Taxes! We encounter so many daily miracles that we now hardly react to them at all. Thanks to our scientists, engineers and technicians, the temperature of our houses is maintained automatically at a pleasant warmth. Well clothed and nourished, we live in luxury: the industrialists are there to interpret our slightest whim, to turn out new products for our comfort and pleasure, endless numbers of 'gadgets' aimed at making our lives ever more comfortable and full of ease. Indeed they invent new requirements for us . . . . Compared to prehistoric time, ours is, in short, a paradise on earth. The Golden Age.

BUT . . . AND THERE IS A BUT . . .

Consider the anonymous multitude passing through our teeming streets, their dejected, anxious faces, their tired, unsmiling features:

their shoulders are hunched, their chests constricted, their stomachs bulge. Civilized maybe, but happy? Most of them are no longer cold nor hungry, but they need pills to send them to sleep, medicine to help evacuate their lazy bowels; they ease their aching heads with aspirin, and swallow tranquillizers to make their lives more bearable. Cut off from nature, we have succeeded amazingly well in polluting the air of our cities, in shutting ourselves into offices and in adulterating our food. The remorseless struggle for money has hardened our hearts, silenced our scruples, and corrupted our moral sense. Mental illness causes more and more havoc every day, while diseases of degeneracy, such as cancer, diabetes and coronary thrombosis, are on the increase, cutting down the flower of our society. The pace of biological degeneration is accelerating to a frightening degree. And yet we are not frightened, we hardly seem aware. Statistics tell us reassuringly that our lifespan has increased by X years, but we do not seem to understand that in just a few generations we are squandering an inheritance built up over hundreds of thousands of years. Civilization, in abolishing the principles of natural selection, allows the survival of defective individuals; while, lapped in luxury, man no longer needs his adaptation mechanism, and his natural defences are thus weakened. How can we stop this degeneration?

Advance in medicine continues daily, but medicine alone is ineffectual. It has accumulated a fund of knowledge which rightly commands our admiration and gives us cause for pride. It has eliminated age-old scourges like plague, smallpox, diphtheria, and countless others besides; it has given us antibiotics, and a whole catalogue of useful remedies, added to every day. Every day, too, our surgeons accomplish new wonders, the heart-transplant operation is only one. But none of this is enough. Rather the reverse; for their very progress in medicine engenders in man a false sense of security. He begins to feel that nothing is forbidden, that no excess is too extreme, that nothing can stand in his way. If he falls ill, all he has to do is to call in the 'Doc', and get him to patch up the damage quickly: it's his job, it's what he's paid for . . . What man will not realize is that his mistaken way of life is responsible for most of his ills, and until he can bring himself to modify it, no doctor however knowledgeable and devoted, can ensure for him anything but a precarious balance of health between this and the next illness. A civilization which culminates in the degeneration of the species, and its individuals, without even granting them some semblance of happiness, must be regarded as having failed.

We are imprisoned by our civilization. What chance have we in the face of such bulldozing? Should we renounce our scientific knowledge? Our technical skills? Our civilized lives? Blow up the factories, burn our books, shut up our scientists, and our technicians? Return to the caves and forest of primeval days?

It is impossible, and it would not help. Besides we are right to be proud of our knowledge and accomplishments. We must not renounce civilization, but make the very best of what it has to give us, and try to minimize its disadvantages.

YOGA: A REMEDY

The solution rests with the individual. But what can he do in isolation—a single being among so many millions? Very little, it would seem. Yet only if each one of us compels himself to follow a strict regime, and yoga is undoubtedly the most practical, effective and best-suited to the demands of modern life, can things change for the better. 'If you wish to change the world, first change yourself.' Thanks to yoga, civilized man can rediscover his zest for life. Yoga bestows on him health and long life, by means of its asanas which give suppleness to the spine—our very life-axis—by calming over-wrought nerves, by relaxing muscles, by reviving organs and nervous centers. Prānayama (the breathing exercises) brings oxygen and energy to every cell, cleanses the organism by burning up waste products, expels the toxins; while relaxation guards against neuras-thenia and insomnia.

The practitioner of yoga looks upon the care of his body as a sacred duty.

Yoga maintains that it is simple to enjoy good health: all that is necessary is to change a few mistaken habits which lead to incalculable ills, misery and premature death. Good health is a birthright: it is as natural to be healthy as it is to be born. Illness originates in neglig-ence, ignorance, or in the flouting of natural laws.

In the yogic sense of the word, illness is a sin of the body: the patient is considered to be as much responsible for his ill-health as he is for any of his wrong actions.

Pyle[1] observed that 'Persons who treat their bodies as they please and transgress rules of personal hygiene of which they should have a

[1] See *A Manual of Personal Hygiene* by W. L. Pyle, A.M., M.D.

definite understanding, are physical sinners. The rules of health are neither restrictive nor straitened. They are in fact simple and few in number and by freeing us from a mass of obstructions which prevent our own strength from acting to the full, and preclude us from the full enjoyment of life, they provide us with a real freedom.' The methods and maxims of yoga, although simple, are also sensible and scientific. So sensible and so easily applied are they that one could be forgiven for wondering how we have come to neglect them so deplorably, thus depriving ourselves of the marvellous benefits which ensue from their regular and careful practice.

The methods described in this book have proved themselves over the course of thousands of years. The author passes on to his readers the yoga tradition which he has been privileged to inherit from his Masters, enriched by his own twenty years of uninterrupted practice. The book is chiefly instructive: it does not stray into theory, but keeps firmly to the field of practice. In the words of Swami Shivananda, 'An ounce of practice is worth several tons of theory'.

2. The Spirit of Hatha-Yoga

Anyone – believer or non-believer – can practice Hatha-yoga success-fully for it is not a religion and it neither demands nor presupposes adherence to any specific philosophy, church or faith. It may be looked upon as a psychosomatic discipline – no more – unique of its kind, unparalleled in its beneficial effects. Since it is essentially a combination of techniques, it is, by definition, a material philosophy, but we should be quite wrong to consider it merely on this technical plane and thereby to ignore the spirit in which it was conceived by the great Sages and Rishis from ancient India – the spirit which gives it its evident quality. No one has defined it more accurately than Swami Shivananda:

'If we acknowledge that man is in truth a spirit incorporated in matter then complete union with Reality must demand the unity of both these aspects. There is much truth in the doctrine which requires man to draw upon what is best from these two worlds. They are in no way incompatible, provided that any action can be seen to conform with the universal laws. The doctrine which avers that happiness in the hereafter may only be found through the absence of joy here on earth must be considered a false philosophy. Happiness and the blessings of Freedom on earth, as in the life beyond, may be attained by approaching every human activity, every duty, in a spirit of adoration. In this way the sadhak (the adept) does not consider himself to be in a state of isolation: he looks upon his life and the interplay of all his activities as integral to it, not to be sought after and guarded jealously for their own sakes, as if joy could be drawn out of life unaided by its own virtue.

'Quite the contrary. Life and all its activities should be regarded as being a part of the sublime action of Nature. The adept can perceive that through his heartbeat is expressed the song of Universal Life. If we ignore the needs of the body, or if we look upon them as ungodly, then we neglect and deny the greatest Life of all of which they are a part, and we falsify the doctrine of the Unity, and the ultimate identity of matter and the Spirit. The humblest of physical needs, when viewed in this light, take on a cosmic significance. The body is Nature; its needs are those of nature: when man rejoices it is Shakti rejoicing through him.

'Everything we do and see, every function of the whole body is evidence of the witness and action of Nature–our mother. If we are fully to appreciate this it is necessary to perfect the manifestation of the body. Man who seeks to become master of himself must accomplish it on every plane–physical, mental and spiritual–since all are interrelated, being but different aspects of the same Universal Consciousness which exists inside him. Who is right? The man who neglects and mortifies his body to obtain a would-be spiritual superiority, or he who cultivates both sides of his character as though different in form from the spirit which moves him? By the techniques of Hatha-yoga, the adept seeks to acquire a perfect body which becomes an instrument sufficient to the harmonious function of mental activity.

'The Hatha-yogi wishes to acquire a body as strong as steel, healthy, free of suffering, ready for long life. He is Master of his body, and would vanquish death. He rejoices in the perfection of his body with its vitality of youth. He would even submit death to his own will, and after his earthly destiny is done, leave this world with one great gesture of dissolution at the hour of his choosing.'

We do not by any means have to accept this doctrine in order to practise Hatha-yoga, but, as well as revealing the state of mind of the true Hatha-yogi, it also dispels certain prejudices widespread in the West, whereby the asanas, for example, are looked upon as stupid acrobatics–useless, even dangerous–and the belief is held that yogis adopt certain painful-looking postures with a view to self-mortification. They may look painful to the uninitiated, but for the trained adept they never induce pain–on the contrary!

3. *To Breathe is to be Alive*

I have seldom seen a man in such distress: he sat before me pale and drawn – his shrunken neck afloat inside the collar of his shirt. He had come, without much conviction, to see me on the advice of a friend – he had problems to explain to me. However, when I say 'explain' do not imagine he confined himself to telling his troubles: his state of exhaustion and nervousness was such that he was almost incoherent. He read aloud from notes he had prepared . . but I will spare you the details. He was married, and a few years previously had suffered some emotional upheaval whose nature he did not disclose. Since then, his health had gradually got worse.

He was suffering from digestive trouble, from palpitations, irritability and lack of concentration. He was growing visibly thinner, losing his zest for life, and was at the end of his tether. He had just changed his job: the pay was better but unfortunately he did not feel able to cope with its new responsibilities. Some important business had to be done next day, and he felt he could not face it. He had decided to hand in his notice.

What was I to do? Exercises were out, for the slightest effort exhausted him. I felt rather inadequate. I wanted to help, but it really did seem that he was not a subject for yoga even in its most elementary form.

In order to help explain this state of affairs, I asked him to take off his coat, lie down on the rug and breathe easily. Because I could see no movement in either stomach or chest, I said to him, 'Don't hold your breath!' 'But I'm not, I'm breathing normally,' came the astonishing reply. Then breathe as deeply as you can.' He made an effort, and his chest rose . . . about half an inch . . . ' I felt his stomach; it was hard and tense. This man was so tense that he was scarcely breathing, only enough to keep himself from suffocation. This explained everything! He looked at me astonished when I told him that he was barely breathing: he had never realized it and nor had anyone else. After half an hour's attempt he succeeded in relaxing a little and breathing through his stomach. The result was in no way remarkable, but, compared with his former state, he was breathing at least five times more air.

Three quarters of an hour later a touch of colour shyly crept into his cheeks, a pale smile lit up his face, and . . . he could speak without his notes. Do not imagine that from now on everything was plain sailing, but through the magic of breathing, a human body had come to life again like a thirsty plant that is being watered. With the help of his doctor, he is now on the way to taking up a normal life.

This is an extreme but not an uninteresting case, and, since this experience, I never fail to lay stress upon the supreme importance of breathing. I notice that, almost without exception, those whose thoracic cage is well developed – and who make full use of it – live without troubles, that is to say they succeed in solving them as and when they arise. Those who breathe badly battle endlessly with problems in every direction: health, profession, emotional life. They are alas, among the majority, for we nearly all breathe more or less badly. How many unfortunate pairs of civilized lungs are never thoroughly ventilated!

Breathing is the great vital source of energy. It is possible to live without solid food for weeks on end, without drink for several days; but without air we die within a few minutes.

Every one of the activities of life is bound up in the processes of oxidation and reduction of carbon dioxide; without oxygen there can be no life.

Our cells depend upon the blood for their supply of oxygen. When the bloodstream in the arteries runs short of oxygen, the vitality of every cell in the body is diminished. It is vital for us to appreciate this first truth: each and every one of the billions of cells in the body are ready to serve you to the utmost. Since each one depends upon its supply of oxygen from that most magic liquid, the blood, you will see how vitally important it is to breathe correctly so that every cell can receive its oxygen.

Not only do we breathe very badly, but often the quality of the air leaves much to be desired, and from this stems our lack of resistance to disease and loss of energy, our unwillingness to perform the slightest physical effort, our nervousness and irritability.

The supply of oxygen is only one aspect of the function of breathing – there is also the elimination of carbon dioxide. The cells have only one way in which to get rid of their waste products – into the blood which is purified by the lungs. What is more, innumerable bacteria may develop in the dark warm humidity of badly-ventilated lungs, so well-suited to their growth. Koch's bacilli cannot withstand the action of oxygen; correct breathing, by ensuring complete ventilation of the lungs, immunizes against tuberculosis.

Of course we didn't have to wait for the Yogis before we could breathe, but in practising their art of breathing you will come to realize just how bad your own has been!

The difference between the breathing habits of the skilled yogi and the uninitiated is as great as between the child floundering in a pool and the champion swimmer. The first battles away, using up a great deal of energy, and in the end can barely keep afloat, the second moves swiftly and effortlessly. The difference lies entirely in the method and its practice.

If only we would learn to breathe properly; the rewards are incalculable!

Swami Shivananda believes strongly in the beneficial effects of yogic respiration: 'The body becomes strong and healthy; excessive fat disappears, the face glows, the eyes are bright and the whole personality radiates a special charm. The voice becomes soft and melodious. The adept is no longer subject to illnesses. The process of digestion is eased, (you will remember how hungry you are after a long walk in the open air). The whole body is purified and the mind improves in its ability to concentrate. Constant practice brings latent spiritual forces to life, and produces happiness and peace.' Before birth the mother breathes for the child, but the level of carbon dioxide in the blood rises at birth and the respiratory apparatus sets off the first and profound indrawn breath. Inside the thoracic cage the lungs unfold and the first independent action is achieved. From now on the ebb and flow of breathing will set the rhythm for life until the last breath is drawn. In the words of C. L. Schleich, from the moment when the midwife cuts the umbilical cord, the lungs are the placenta which binds man to the cosmic mother.

To be alive is to breathe – to breathe is to be alive. Yogis measure by the number of respirations the length of human life.

Before we undertake any complicated breathing exercises, let us first learn to breathe well. Rather let us re-learn . . . for we all once knew it in infancy . . . Many things in our lives have changed since then, and not always for the better, particularly in this matter of breathing, which has often become an incomplete, superficial, gasping, sometimes hasty procedure. This is because we are perpetually tense, wrought up, prey to negative emotions; anxiety, anger and much else.

Before we can improve our breathing we must remember that the process existed long before we did—we have nothing to teach it. What we have to do is to prepare ourselves to receive its revitalizing strength by removing any obstacles that might hinder its good effects. Proper breathing depends on our eliminating tension, correcting bad habits, wrong mental and physical attitudes; the moment we get rid of these obstacles it will come into its own and bring us vitality and good health.

The corsets of 1900 are no longer in fashion, but there is still more than one item of clothing which prevents us from normal breathing—leather belts for men, girdles and brassières for women. These must be as flexible as possible if they are not to hinder respiration.

But the physical obstacles are even more daunting: the hard tense stomach which encumbers every breath, imprisoning the personality; the rib-cage as inflexible as a breast-plate; the diaphragm immobilized by the wind—itself caused by spasms—which has accumulated in the alimentary canal. The first step is to relax all these muscles, which when permanently tense are designed more successfully than any corset to prevent normal breathing; and this is why relaxation is the open door to yoga.

PRIORITY GIVEN TO EXHALATION

In the act of respiration, Westerners give precedence to the in-drawing of the breath. Yoga, on the other hand, maintains that all good respiration begins with a slow and complete *exhalation,* and that this perfect exhalation is an absolute prerequisite of correct and complete inhalation, for the very simple reason that, until a receptacle is emptied, it cannot be filled. Unless we first breathe out fully it is impossible to breathe in correctly.

Normal respiration therefore, begins with a slow calm exhalation carried out by relaxing of the inspiratory muscles. The chest is depressed by its own weight, expelling the air. This out breath must be as silent as every other action involved in breathing (you should not hear yourself breathe), and because it is silent, it will also be *slow*. At the end of the expiration the abdominal muscles help the lungs to empty to their fullest extent, by means of a contraction which expels the last traces of tainted air. The spongy make-up of the lungs does not allow them to be emptied completely—there is always a residue of impure air in the lungs. We must attempt to minimize this 'residue' because together with the fresh air provided by inhalation it makes up the actual air we breathe. The more complete the exhalation, therefore, the greater the quantity of fresh air to enter the lungs, and so the purer the air in contact with the alveolar surfaces.

The total volume of air which the lungs are able to contain is known as 'the vital capacity'. A more apt term cannot be imagined, and innumerable techniques have been thought up aimed at increasing this capacity. Before we can contemplate this improvement we must make use of what we already possess by carefully exhaling. Yoga recognizes three separate forms of breathing: diaphragmatic, intercostal and clavicular. Complete yogic breathing combines all three, and constitutes the ideal technique.

Diaphragmatic Breathing
The majority of men breathe in this way. The diaphragm subsides while the breath is being drawn in, and the abdominal region swells. This is the least faulty method of breathing. The base of the lungs fills with air, and the rhythmic lowering of the diaphragm produces a constant, gentle massage of the whole abdominal content, and helps these organs to function correctly.

Intercostal Breathing
This is achieved by raising the ribs through dilating the thoracic cage or chest wall like a pair of bellows. It is a form of breathing which fills the middle section of the lungs, allowing less air to enter than in abdominal respiration, and more important, involving far more effort! This is 'athletic' respiration. When combined with abdominal breathing it ventilates the lungs satisfactorily.

Clavicular Breathing
Air is introduced by raising the collar-bone and shoulders. In this way, only the upper part of the lungs receives any fresh air. It is the least satisfactory method of breathing and is often characteristic of women.

Complete Breathing
Complete yogic respiration incorporates all three methods, integrated into one single, full and rhythmic movement.

The method is best studied while you are lying on your back, here is a brief description of the various phases:

(1) Empty the lungs entirely.
(2) Slowly lower the diaphragm allowing air to enter the lungs. When the abdomen swells filling the bottom of the lungs with air . . .
(3) . . . expand the ribs without straining, then . . .
(4) . . . allow the lungs to fill completely by raising the collar-bones.

Throughout the procedure, the air should enter in a continuous flow, without gasping. No noise must be made for it is essential to breathe silently[1].

It is of the utmost importance to concentrate the mind entirely upon the action of breathing.

When the lungs are completely filled, breathe out, in the same sequence as when inhaling. Now breathe in again in the same way. You may continue for as long as you wish. It should not induce any discomfort or fatigue. You can practise it at any time of day, whenever you think of it, at work, walking, any time; breathe consciously and as completely as possible. Gradually you will acquire the habit of complete respiration, and your method of breathing will improve as you go on. It is essential to reserve daily, for a few minutes' practice, a special time convenient to yourself (the morning when you wake up is a good time, and so is the evening before going to sleep).

Whenever you feel tired, depressed or discouraged do a few complete breathing exercises; your fatigue will disappear magically, your mental balance will be re-established and you will set to work again with renewed will.

Inspiration like exhalation must be silent, slow, continuous and easy. Do not blow yourself up like a balloon or a tyre. Breathe easily without straining. Remember that the ideal respiration is *deep, slow, silent, easy.* Those engaged in sedentary work are liable to accumulations of blood or to develop congestion in one organ or another. The slowing down of the bloodstream produces wear and premature ageing in the organism. With complete breathing, the bloodstream in our organs is prevented from slowing down to the

---

[1] Details of this complete breathing will be given in the following chapter.

point where it stagnates and degenerates from 'stream' into 'marsh'.

One of the most important correlations between deep respiration and circulation is the effect, induced by deep breathing, of suction, of aspiration. The technical reason is given in an example by Dr Fritsche.

The large vein continuously pouring blood from the liver into the heart is emptied regularly through suction developed by the lungs in breathing. When the venous blood from the liver fails to circulate freely the liver swells and becomes congested and this has unfortunate repercussions on the circulation of the blood which supplies the alimentary canal, which in turn can cause digestive trouble.

Deep, slow breathing is capable of dispersing almost instantaneously this condition of congestion in the liver, for *the lungs literally suck up* the excess blood accumulated in the liver, and pour it into the right auricle (side of the heart). Moreover *the movements made by the diaphragm and thoracic cage have the effect of accelerating the venous circulation throughout the organism.*

When you breathe in, not only do you inhale *air* into the lungs but at the same time *blood* is pumped through every tissue in the body. According to research made by P. Heger, when the lungs are completely filled with air they contain the maximum amount of blood.

When, therefore, the diaphragm is depressed and flattened during the first phase of breathing, the inferior *vena cava,* because its walls are contracting, propels its blood towards the heart.

Deep slow breathing is, therefore, a powerful driving force in circulation. The heart is the forcing-pump propelling the blood into the arterial network, while the lungs act as a suction-pump on the venous circulation. Circulation depends upon the correct interaction of these two driving forces. It is the finest tonic of all for the heart.

The optimum interchange of gases in the lung, the absorption of oxygen, and the giving off of carbon dioxide are most satisfactory when breathing is deep, complete and *slow*. According to Walter Michel: 'If the ventilation of the lungs is not complete, plentiful and slow, the surfaces to be oxygenated suffer in performance, and the fixation of oxygen is incompletely carried out even when ferments are present.'

It is essential for this optimum gaseous interchange that 'the venous blood adapt its tension *slowly* to the alveolar air . . . When alveolar air remains for long in contact with the blood, the maximum degree of union is effected – i.e. after the aerated blood has remained for ten to twenty seconds in the alveoli. The rate of blood circulation and the length of time during which the air remains in the alveoli–in other words the degree of capacity and the *method of respiration being used*–play an equal part in determining the quantity of the interchanges of gases in the lungs. Through deep inspiration and by retention of the air breathed in, the diffusion surface is increased. The effective surface is also increased, since all the normally inactive alveoli unused in everyday breathing, are brought into service. Thus medical practice is justified in concluding that correct filling of the alveoli is necessary to complete oxygenation. It is essential that the greatest possible number of alveoli take part in the process, so that the surface covered is increased. According to physiologists it is also necessary for the air breathed in to remain for ten to twenty seconds in the alveoli in order to obtain as complete an interchange of the respiratory gases as can be attained . . .' This illustrates how essential rhythm is in breathing, and especially to what an extent *slow* breathing affects the respiration of the tissues, which by this simple device, increases more than in any other way the available consumption supply of oxygen throughout the organism.

'Every organic or functional disorder leading to conditions of illness is susceptible to the influence, if not always the cure, of controlled breathing.'

'Potential bronchitic, asthmatic and emphysematic patients are invariably cases who breathe insufficiently', says Dr Peschier.

'Controlled respiration is the most outstanding method known to us for increasing organic resistance. Reduce the organic resistance by any means whatsoever and you will see germs, which up to that moment have been non-injurious, now developing into agents of infection [Pasteur]. There are failures in the use of serotherapy by sulphonamides, as well as by penicillin: certain remedies like these have no direct action on the infectious agent. On the other hand, it is known that certain states of the blood or of fluids in the tissues (temperature, density, viscous state or simply pH degree) are enough to destroy an infection without the help of any therapy from outside.

'There is a natural immunity attributed to an ionic balance in the blood, and dependent upon breathing, which, in acting upon the pH in the tissue-fluids, reacts upon the optimum pH content of the microbe. It confers on the balance of the acid-base a regularity which is re-established with each breath, allowing the organism to maintain or recover its vital pH.

'If controlled breathing is not always sufficient to combat infectious illnesses, it at least supports the struggle which rids us of them, and provides the organism with ways of avoiding them.'

The foresight of the yogis who, thousands of years ago, established the rules and methods of ideal breathing is astonishing! They advised us to breathe as though at our birth we had been allotted a certain number of respirations, and our lives would last until this capital 'number of respirations' came to an end. Had we inherited this belief, how careful would we be to breathe slowly. There is no doubt that to breathe is to live. But to breathe slowly is to live long – and to enjoy good health.

While it is necessary to practice asanas on an empty stomach, and to wear suitable clothing and choose an appropriate place, controlled breathing may be practised anywhere, at any time, without attracting the notice of even our most immediate companions!

Begin the day with some deep, slow, silent breaths while you lie in bed in the few minutes before you get up . . . And, all through your asana session, breathe in the yogic manner. If you have to walk home from work, breathe in the same way! Breathe in for six steps as you walk, then hold the breath for three, finally exhaling it to the count of twelve steps. As a general rule, exhalation should last for twice as long as inspiration, whether or not you hold your breath. You can begin with, say: four steps for inspiration, two for holding the breath, and eight for letting it go.

During the day, at work or elsewhere, each time you remember – often, let us hope – take time off for a few deep, complete, slow breaths, and during the evening take a moment off for a short session of breathing in bed – this will probably lull you to sleep. You may continue to breathe in the same rhythm that you used when walking, but perhaps this time counting the seconds.

In this way by an accumulation of short but frequent sessions during the day, you are ensuring for yourself the incalculable advantages of yogic breathing.

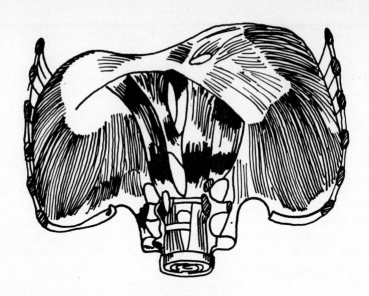

THE DIAPHRAGM SEEN FROM BELOW

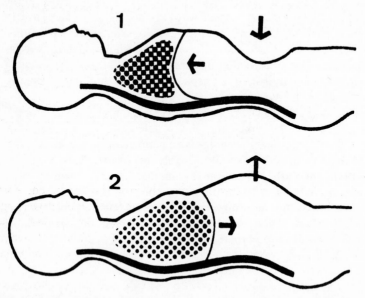

SKETCH SHOWING POSITION OF DIAPHRAGM WITH (1) EMPTIED
LUNGS (2) FILLED LUNGS.

4. *Complete Yogic Respiration*

This chapter is a summary of the technique of complete yogic respiration: it is the only standard one, in that it incorporates in a single action the various partial methods of breathing. Let us first summarize what we have already learned.

Inhalation is made up of three partial phases:

(a) abdominal breathing induced by lowering and flattening the dome-shaped diaphragm.
(b) intercostal breathing brought about by expanding the ribs.
(c) clavicular breathing from the top of the lungs, produced by raising the upper part of the thorax.

Each of these phases has its own merits, but yogic inspiration is only complete when all three are done in conjunction.
How can this breathing be learnt?

In the first place, before attempting to combine them – that is to say before we can achieve in one single, smooth and continuous movement complete and easy filling of the lungs, thereby supplying them with reviving air, and expanding the pulmonary alveoli (all 70 million of them) – we must learn to dissociate the three phases. First of all we practise breathing from the diaphragm.

DIAPHRAGMATIC BREATHING
In order to learn to breathe correctly from the diaphragm – easily completely and naturally – it is wise to practise it lying down, since it is then easier to relax the muscles of the abdominal wall, which served to hold us upright when we are sitting or walking. Later you will be able to breathe from the diaphragm whenever required – even when walking or running.

To ensure complete comfort it is often a good idea to place a cushion under the knees: this diminishes the lumbar arch. Do not lie on too soft a surface, because although it is possible to breathe from the diaphragm when in bed, it is even better to do the exercises on some firm support–such as a rug laid on the floor.

When practising it is a good idea to close the eyes: this helps to increase concentration.

Before you begin, be sure to breathe out completely a few times; either by giving a few sighs, after which you pull in the stomach thus contracting the abdominal muscles, in order to get rid of any remaining air, or, if alone in the room, by emitting the sound OM (see page 42). This obliges you to breathe out slowly and completely– and since the sound should be uniform, you will be able to expel the remainder of the air at the rate required. Sound a long and sonorous OOOOOMMMMM, vibrating the MMMM inside the skull, and concentrating meanwhile upon the various muscles of which the abdomen is composed. After a few long, slow, deep exhalations there is an automatic tendency to breathe in more deeply from the stomach. We are going to try to accentuate this tendency as far as possible. The first sketch shows the position of the diaphragm when the lungs are empty. You will see that it has risen very high up in the thoracic cage like a piston in a cylinder, and the lungs occupy a very restricted space. It is important to empty the lungs thoroughly, thereby getting rid of the greatest possible amount of air. This piston-like structure is however not rigid, and unlike that of a motor-car is not flat, but convex rather like the lid of a casserole (see sketch 2). The diaphragm has a rather rigid, flat central section–the aponeurotic– and is surrounded by a girdle of peripheral muscles whose contraction determines its downward movements: the diaphragm muscles are among the strongest in the human body, or perhaps we should say, they are designed to be the strongest, because their owner alas, may allow them to atrophy. From sketch 1 we can also understand why complete relaxation is only possible once the lungs are emptied without forcible exhalation–because at that moment the diaphragm muscles are at rest.

Absolute relaxation, therefore can only exist during those few seconds of respite which we allow when we hold our breath with the *lungs empty*.

Having completely emptied the lungs and held the breath for a few seconds, you will soon realize that your breathing is attempting to start up *on its own*–therefore relax your stomach and allow the breath to flow. As air enters the lungs, the stomach expands and rises, because the dome of the diaphragm has flattened, and *not because the muscles in the abdominal region have contracted.* People believe, often in all good faith, that they are 'breathing from the stomach', because they are flexing their abdominal muscles. In fact, the latter should be relaxed, and must remain so throughout the inhalation. The lungs gradually fill with air from beneath. The inhalation will be slow, easy and unquestionably silent. If you do not hear yourself breathing it means that your respiration has acquired the correct slowness. If audible it means you have inhaled with too much haste.

It is essential to breathe in as well as out through the nose.

The stomach should rise gently like a balloon being blown up, and the muscle structure should remain supple: should you wish to control the movement you may place your hand on your stomach near the navel, at the same time resting the elbow on the floor. In this way it is easy to follow the expanding movement of the stomach. While this is going on, place the other hand against one side so that you can ensure that the ribs remain completely still, and so realize that abdominal and thoracic breathing are completely separate.

Should your ribs still move while the stomach is rising, they should be immobilized by girding the thorax with a belt placed near the lower part of the sternum, in the pit of the stomach. Fasten the belt when the lungs are empty, to the required girth. While you breathe in, the ribs will meet resistance from the belt and will take no part in the breathing and your diaphragm will be forced to flatten and your stomach to expand.

While you are breathing in, you should be conscious of what is going on in the warm depths of the thorax; you will soon find you are conscious of the movements of the diaphragm, and you will be able to separate the two phases and dispense with the belt.

The Effects of Diaphragmatic Breathing
This method of breathing is both relaxing and one of the most active of the forces which drive the circulation. The diaphragm is truly our 'second heart', of which the piston-like movements expand the base of the lungs, enabling them to suck in a great quantity of venous blood. The venous circulation being accelerated, the heart is well supplied with blood from the back, as already described, and this definitely improves the general circulation.

The down-and-up movement of this diaphragmatic piston also

gives a very helpful massage – gentle yet powerful – to the abdominal organs.

The liver becomes decongested and the gall-bladder evacuates the bile as required. The increased rate of circulation in the liver and the gall-bladder prevents stones forming in the bladder. The spleen, stomach, pancreas, kidneys, and the entire digestive tract, are massaged and toned up. Stasis of the blood is eliminated – it is quite usual to hear some gurgling sounds when practising diaphragmatic breathing, and this shows that the peristaltic movements of the digestive tract are being activated.

With practice, this abdominal breathing becomes progressively more complete, supple, relaxed and rhythmic, where at the outset it was jerky and difficult in certain subjects – the very tense person for example.

Note here the decongestant action of this breathing on the solar plexus – the abdominal vegetative brain (it is important to emphasize this), whose significance (sometimes its very existence) is often completely ignored. It is also the 'plexus of anxiety' and this explains the calming, peaceful effect which abdominal breathing has upon it.

As a rule, men learn this form of breathing much more easily than women, who should not be put off from attempting it.

BREATHING FROM THE RIBS

We are now going to learn thoracic or costal breathing.

As its name implies, this is the action of expanding the thorax which leads to the inflation of the lungs by conducting air into them. This time we work sitting in a chair or on the ground, it does not matter which. Empty the lungs completely and keep the abdominal muscles contracted: in this way it becomes impossible to breathe through the stomach. Throughout the inhalation you should keep the stomach contracted in order to prevent any breathing through the diaphragm.

Needless to say those who used a belt to keep the ribs from moving, should remove it for learning thoracic breathing!

Place the hands on the sides a few inches away from the armpits, in such a way that the palms can feel the ribs. Point the fingers to the front. Breathe in, attempting at the same time to push out the hands as far as possible with the ribs, that is, not in front of you but towards the sides. After a few attempts, you will feel the exact position.

You will notice clearly a greater resistance to the entrance of air than you did during the abdominal breathing, which allowed entry to the largest volume of air with a minimum of effort.

Despite this resistance a fairly large quantity of air will enter during thoracic inhalation.

Breathe about twenty times from the ribs only.

CLAVICULAR OR HIGH BREATHING

In this type of breathing, you must attempt to raise the collar-bones while air is being inhaled.

Immobilize the abdominal muscles, in the same way as you did when you were learning thoracic breathing, and keep the hands upon the sides in the position described previously. Now try to allow the air to enter by drawing the collar-bones up towards the chin, without however raising the shoulders, which will anyhow be almost impossible if the hands are kept on the sides.

You will feel air entering, but you will also be aware that a very small quantity does so, despite a considerably greater effort than that involved in thoracic breathing.

This is the least efficient way of breathing, but women habitually do it. If you watch women breathing, eight out of ten will show no signs of breathing other than a distinct raising of the collar-bone, while their brooches or necklaces rise and fall. This is a form of breathing used also by nervous subjects and those suffering from a degree of debility or anxiety. It is only useful or to be tolerated when it is integrated into complete yogic breathing, and only takes on meaning when it is preceded by the two other phases of this breathing.

Why Do Women Breathe from the Top of the Lungs?

For a long time it was thought that the restrictions of clothing such as corsets, belts, brassières, and other tightly-fitting clothes were solely responsible. However even women who do not wear corsets – these mercifully are tending to disappear and modern belts are very flexible – use this type of breathing even when their clothes are no more constricting than mens. We feel we should look further for the deeper reasons behind this state of affairs.

When babies of both sexes have been observed it has been noted that breast-fed females, although breathing for the greater part of the time through the stomach in the same way as their male counterparts, have moments when their breathing is carried out through

33

the apex of the chest. In these cases it can hardly be clothing that is responsible! To find the answer, we should look at the fundamental role which differentiates the female from the male; her ability to bear children.

What happens during pregnancy? As the uterus increases in size, it invades the abdominal cavity and during the later months of pregnancy the mother is virtually unable to breathe any longer from the diaphragm, since this now cannot be lowered owing to the presence of the child and the placenta. The woman then falls back on the emergency method provided; and this is clavicular breathing. If you watch a pregnant woman you will see that she is forced to breathe in this way particularly in the last weeks of the pregnancy. Deep breathing for her is clearly impossible. The female baby is training from the cradle instinctively to understand and practise this sort of respiration.

Let us, however, return to the subject of clothing and the part it plays. As soon as an article of clothing compresses the abdomen, however little, the defence mechanism starts up, and the woman breathes from the top of the chest, whereas in similar circumstances men react differently, by loosening their clothes, or in managing somehow despite the obstruction to lower the diaphragm – that is they fight the obstacle, whereas women bypass it.

It is nevertheless true that this form of breathing is inferior in quality to abdominal respiration, and women should avoid using it habitually, since it is a type of breathing provided for use in very specific circumstances. Clearly, then, women must guard against using this method of breathing except when pregnant.

LEARN COMPLETE YOGIC BREATHING

Yogic breathing as we know, incorporates the three types of partial respiration.

In the first stages of learning, it is best to lie flat on the back. Begin by breathing slowly and deeply from the stomach, and, when you feel that it is impossible to raise the stomach any further, expand the ribs, and allow still more air to enter the lungs. When the ribs are fully extended, raise the collar-bones so that yet a little more air can enter. By this time you are filled to the brim with air. (You should not, however, blow yourself up like a balloon; the whole process should remain easy and comfortable.) Avoid any tensing of the muscles of the hands, face and neck, particularly in the last stage

34

(clavicular) of the breathing. The three movements, as we have already pointed out, should be done in a 'chain link' system, keeping them entirely separate and visible to the outside observer.

FAULTS: Having allowed the stomach to fill with air by flattening the diaphragm, people sometimes cut short the entry of air at that moment, drawing in the stomach in order to allow the air to rise (or so they think) to the apex of the lungs.

GIDDINESS

Occasionally people who breathe habitually through the apex of the lungs find that complete yogic respiration brings on a feeling of giddiness–completely harmless in itself, but somewhat unpleasant. How does this occur? It is simply the effect of suction which is literally aspirating the venous blood, notably from the brain, which is nothing but beneficial. If the subject suffers from slightly low blood pressure this slight fall in inter-cerebral blood pressure induces the feeling just described. The remedy is very simple; the legs should be raised to the vertical position–that is to say at right angles to the trunk, as you are lying down; the blood pressure will at once be re-established, and the giddiness vanishes. Should the exercises be continued? Absolutely, since in a few days the organism adapts itself, and this slight and harmless inconvenience will disappear.

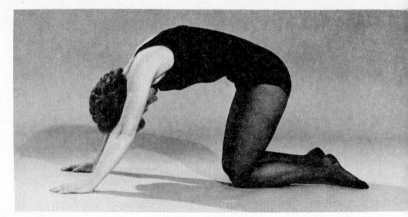

This exercise, which is completely straightforward, teaches control of the abdominal muscles during breathing, which restores all latent mobility to the diaphragm.

The above illustration shows the first position to be taken up: Emptying the lungs completely, arch the spine, look towards the navel, and contract the stomach in order to expel the last traces of air. In this way the exhalation is active.

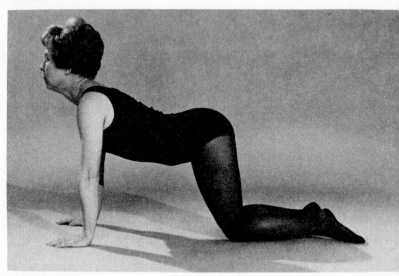

The inspiration which succeeds it is *passive*. It is made by relaxing the muscular part of the abdomen so that air enters effortlessly into the lungs. Accentuate the breathing-in movement by hollowing the back, and looking up. Repeat these two stages ten times, then continue practising, this time lying down.

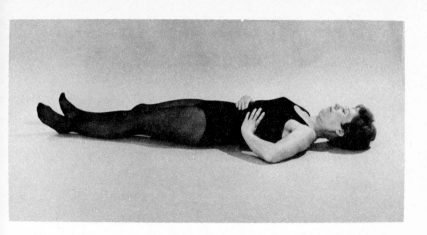

Place one hand over the hollow part of the stomach, the other over one side. The adept will be able to pick out clearly the various movements made in breathing. This photograph shows the final phase of exhalation. The stomach is drawn in to expel the last trace of air, while the ribs contract.

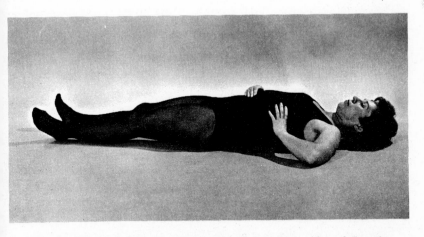

Throughout the breathing-in process the hands have been able to follow the abdominal phase, the rib phase and finally the clavicular phase of yogic breathing. At the end of the inhalation, the thorax is found to be filled with air, as the photograph shows, but the stomach is not blown out especially in the area below the navel.

5. *Goodbye to Colds*

Yogis have devised various procedures by means of which the organism may be purified and kept scrupulously clean. To some extent, the body disposes of residues and toxins spontaneously: the kidneys filter the blood and we throw off in urination the very toxic uric content; the intestines remove from the body any remains after digestion has been completed; the skin also throws off toxins while the lungs get rid of an excess of carbon dioxide. Yoga supports these organs while they carry out their tasks, and aids Nature in its cleansing work, since there are certain waste products which the body is unable to throw off automatically. This is why we have to wash our skin daily, clean our teeth, and so on. But yoga goes very much further.

Let us look first at the Neti technique of 'the nasal douche' which is neither difficult nor disagreeable.

To breathe is to live, but to breathe well your nose must be clean. Mucus is secreted in order to capture the dust content in the air before it reaches the lungs: minute vibrating hairs move in the opposite direction to the air and collect these particles of dust. When we blow our noses, we get rid of a large proportion of this mucus, but yogis do not regard this as sufficient. The nasal douche, Neti, cleans in depth the mucous membrane of the nose which is highly stocked with nerves, and by way of reflex it is possible to affect the function of organs which are often very remote. You may remember that there is a medical technique known as 'endonasal reflexotherapy' which is a form of healing by titillating certain nerve endings of the mucous membrane in the nose. In any case, Neti cleans it thoroughly.

The olfactory nerve also benefits from this douche, and so do the eyes, since it activates the circulation of blood in the nasal fossae. In addition, Neti guards against head-colds, for which no specific cure has yet been discovered.

The technique is simple. A bowl full of tepid salted water is all that is necessary. For certain osmotic reasons water without salt may cause pricking. A teaspoon of salt added to the water will re-establish the osmotic balance. If the water can be boiled so much the better.

Hold the bowl horizontally and plunge the nostrils into the water.

Do not breathe in the water as you would breathe in air; it would enter too violently; use the epiglottis to make little pumping movements in the back of the throat. The water will move up the nose without your feeling it, until after a few pumping movements you taste the salt entering your throat. Make sure that air does not get in at the same time as the water. Stop breathing in, wait a few seconds, keeping the nostrils in the water, and then allow the water itself to run out of the nose. Repeat the whole operation. After three irrigations (more if you wish), a few strong exhalations with each nostril blocked in turn, will expel the remains of any water from the passages of the nose. That's all! Just try, and observe the results!

6. *Tongue Dhauti*

The most intensive regard to cleanliness of the body is essential to Hatha-yogis, and is one of the foundations of good health. Our view of hygiene agrees, but it is limited to externals, while in yoga complete internal cleanliness is sought after. As a result, there are methods of purification which, it must be admitted, are rejected by Westerners, and even cause them a certain apprehension or disgust. I will not therefore deal with stomach or colonic irrigations, though they are in fact more frightening in imagination than in reality.

We will confine ourselves to the cleaning of the tongue, which is practised little in the West.

Our ordinary methods of hygiene neglect that active organ. Some people, however, do clean their tongue with a toothbrush. The intention behind this is good but the method mistaken, for the bristles irritate the tongue, and do little good, while it is easy with the handle of the brush to damage the very delicate structure of the soft palate.

The yogic method uses a tongue-scraper or scratcher made of wood. A coffee-spoon will serve instead. Turn the convex part upwards, and scrape the tongue with the edge. After a few movements from back to front, examine the spoon; you will be convinced of the need for the operation! Scrape the tongue once more from left to right and vice versa, stopping only when the spoon no longer yields any impurities, then, in front of the looking-glass make the expressive although undistinguished gesture of sticking out your tongue, and look . . . how clean and pink it is!

Why do yogis lay so much stress on the cleanness of the tongue? First on the principle of cleanliness itself: furthermore they consider that the tongue is the tool which absorbs prāna (energy in subtle form) from food. As long as there is any taste in food it contains prāna. The taste buds fulfil important functions which we will not go into here: they work especially through reflex action, in close collaboration with the salivary glands: the more delicious the food, the more abundant is salivation. Effective salivation of food is of the utmost importance, notably because of the presence of ptyaline, a very active ferment contained in the saliva, which, among other things, acts on starches and pre-digests food. But the results of the stimulation to the taste buds are not limited to the salivary glands: the stomach, thus warned, prepares itself for work. In short, by way of reflex action, the stimulation of the taste buds influences the entire digestive system. If the tongue is 'burdened', the taste buds are coated, mucous matter making them viscous, so that tastes will not be enjoyed so acutely in their full freshness, and stimulus will be much reduced. Finally a coated tongue will sometimes cause bad breath. How many times a day should a tongue be scraped? Once or twice is enough; a good moment is when the teeth are cleaned. This should become a sensible habit – nothing more.

7. *OM*

So said the Swami of Chidambaram to Yeats-Brown, the author of *Bengal Lancer* –

'Repeat internally the basic sound which I now give you as your word of power, OM. Concentrate on this word which has been from the beginning . . .'

'How concentrate?' Yeats-Brown asked; 'OM has no very definite meaning for me. It seems a pleasant sound, but nothing more!'

'It need be nothing more at present. Concentrate your mind on Its pleasant sound. You know that we consider It to be the Word by which the worlds were made, the root of language, and the end of vision. However, It will work in your Unconscious whether you like It or dislike It: It need not be intellectualized, and I need not go into Its symbolism.'[1]

Swami Chidambaram's words indicate the overwhelming importance which yogis give to this mysterious vocable 'OM'.

It is heard very little among Western practitioners of yoga, but in India – in fact throughout the whole of Asia – this syllable is heard wherever one goes. 'OM', together with the scent of dhoop (an incense with a sandalwood base), pervades the ashrams, temples and caves. In India OM is sacred, which is doubtless the reason why in the West we have failed to give it its rightful place in our practice of yoga.

Roman Catholics tend to mistrust it, fearing to participate in some 'pagan' ritual which might lead them into heresy; the unbeliever merely sees it as a superstition and turns away with a shrug.

And yet OM is a unique sound: If repeated regularly, far from being an absurd or useless practice, it has many good effects on the physical side as well as upon the mind; it deserves objective examination before being – if need be – discarded as a practice.

I have looked in vain into many books devoted to yoga for some

[1] Taken from *Lancer at Large* by the same author.

rational explanation of its effects. I therefore looked for help in un-prejudiced experience, common sense and the knowledge given to us by Western science. However, let us learn first of all to form the sound of 'OM': Lying down or sitting, lips apart, breathe in very deeply, then exhale, slowing down the expulsion of the breath which in its passage, causes the vocal chords to vibrate in a prolonged sound of 'Oo . . .' continued until the lungs are almost completely emptied. The sound should be made as weightily and evenly as possible. If properly made, with the hand laid flat over the thorax (sternum), you should feel some vibration in the neighbourhood of the collar-bone. At the end of the exhalation, close the mouth and, by contracting the stomach muscles to expel the remnants of air, make a deep humming sound, which will seem to reverberate in the cranium. The other hand, laid on the top of the head, should also sense the vibration.

If you apply the palms of your hands to your ears, you will hear the 'O . . . m' even more clearly.

And now for the effects which this practice will produce:

1. *The Effects of the Vibrations*
The 'O . . .' vibrates through the whole bone structure of the thoracic cage, which proves that the vibration reaches down to the air in the lungs, and that the delicate membrane of the alveoli in contact with the air must also vibrate, stimulating the pulmonary cells and allow-ing a better exchange of gases. Recent works of Western physiolo-gists assure us that this vibration also produces very significant effects upon the endocrine glands, the importance of which is increasingly being stressed by science. Dr Leser-Lasario, indeed. devoted twenty-five years of his life as a scientist to the study of the effects produced in the human organism by vocal vibrations. His efforts established scientifically and beyond doubt that the sounding of vocables during exhalation automatically massages the organs by vibrations. These vibrations reach the deep-lying tissues and nerve cells; the circulation of blood increases in the tissues and organs involved. The ductless glands, which pour hormones directly into the blood and lymph, are stimulated (the pituitary, pineal, thyroid, thymus, supra-renal and gonads). These vibrations also benefit the sympathetic system and the vagus nerve. The muscular structure of the respiratory apparatus is at the same time relaxed and strengthened. Breathing improves, and with it the provision of

oxygen to the whole body. The organs in the thoracic cage and the abdomen are particularly subject to the effect of the vibro-massage which the sound 'O . . .' induces. Electro-magnetic waves are produced by the vibrations, which multiply all through the body, increasing energy and *joie de vivre*. Concentration is improved (see 'Mental effects' below, p. 45). Leser-Lasario's experiments have proved that the entire body relaxes under the influence of this internal vibro-massage, which frees inhibitions and reduces depressions and inferiority complexes, unifying or integrating the whole psyche. After all, it is only through vibrations that music produces the most complex emotions in us.

The humming reverberates in the head causing the cranial nerves to vibrate.

2. *Slow Exhalation*
By making the sound 'Oo . . .' the rate of exhalation is slowed down: you already know how beneficial this slow breathing is.

3. *Regular Exhalation*
When the sound is uniform throughout the exhalation, the latter is not only slow, but regular and smooth.

4. *Complete Exhalation*
The chapter devoted to breathing has demonstrated the importance of slow and total exhalation, in expelling the maximum of vitiated air from the lungs and reducing to the utmost the volume of residual air. When you have finished sounding OM, you can be certain that your lungs have been emptied to the maximum degree. This complete emptying has an immediate effect on inhalation, which likewise becomes full and deep.

5. *Control and Relaxation of the Respiratory System*
Exhalation is produced through the relaxation of the muscles of the respiratory system. If the exhalation is to be uniform it is essential that this relaxation be controlled. Where there is tension around the throat or in the muscles of the thoracic cage, the sound emitted is jerky. Continuous, smooth sound indicates that there is complete control and mastery of the progressive relaxation of every muscle

in the respiratory apparatus, and this leads to the elimination of unconscious tensions, and ensures that the inhalation which follows is easy and flexible.

6. *Mental Effects*
The effects of 'OM' on the mind are no less important than on the body. Let us remember first that the civilized brain-worker's mind is primarily full of words. Quite apart from speech or reading, we talk to ourselves inwardly; we form sentences in the mind, rather than pictures. If you observe yourself you will see just how far the words in your mind have suppressed the mental image. Yet since mental images are dynamic, the *visual* faculty is a prime necessity for control of the mind, for learning the art of thinking and for acquiring certain powers within yourself. Further, there is a close connection between the mechanism of the brain in forming sentences and the mechanism of speech, which involves an enormous expenditure of nervous energy.

Speech represents power: many great men have also been great orators. Let us eliminate futile verbiage – the blah-blah-blah – for the result is a great and immediate economy of nervous energy. In other words we are left with a greater amount of energy available for other tasks.

While the air is slowly leaving your lungs and causing your vocal cords to vibrate, listen carefully to the long 'Oom' and note that it fills the entire field of consciousness and that meanwhile the processes engaged in forming sentences are inhibited.

After a troublesome day this is a marvellous way to dispel ferment in yourself and reinduce calm.

The sound 'Om' can by its nature only be made audibly by exhaling: however when you breathe in you can listen to it mentally. You will not get any of the results (1–5) just described, but on the other hand your mind will become much calmer. When circumstances do not permit you to vocalize the syllable, then repeat it to yourself internally, and the same favourable results to the mind will ensue. Repeat 'Om' often during the day silently in your mind and experience the calm and the peace which it brings.

8. *Relaxation*

Tense, overwrought, nervous and anxious, modern man is caught up in the hellish grind which drives him inexorably into 'stress', because his constant state of anxiety prevents him from facing up to the relentless demands of modern life which, behind an amiable and comfortable exterior, conceals an inhuman machine and an unrelenting struggle for existence. Is it really surprising, then, that millions of civilized beings live with the depressing feeling that they are 'out of step', overlaid by apparently impossible tasks with which they cannot possibly cope, and from which they can never escape? Tranquillizers, the 'happy' pills of modern chemistry, do bring an apparent respite; but in the long run the cure is worse than the disease, since it does no more than damp down the roots of this anxiety and nervousness without eradicating them. But there are two sorts of remedy, both preventive and curative: controlled breathing and relaxation. The latter is the most direct antidote.

What is more, relaxation is essential to true yoga and without it there is no chance of happiness, peace or health. The tense person, even when he has everything to make him happy, keeps happiness at arm's length. Finally – and this is by no means the least of its virtues – relaxation is the source of creative thought. As Cicero said: 'Only the man who can relax is able to create, and ideas reach his mind like lightning.'

Relaxation in the midst of action should not be the exclusive prerogative of small children and animals (the cat is a model example); we should all learn once more to relax our bodies consciously every day for a few minutes, so that we remain relaxed thereafter in any situation. We must first however, understand the underlying techniques so as to grasp their purpose and apply them intelligently. Then we can study the methods which lead towards this deliciously restful state which is better than sleep itself. The art of relaxation can be acquired, and those experiencing the euphoria it brings for the first time find in it a revelation. The body which had become lifeless and heavy is cast off limp and relaxed, while the spirit seems to soar, freed from material affairs, outside its earthly shell.

We shall now look for a moment into the subject of anatomy, leaving aside specialized detail. There are two types of muscle – first the voluntary ones attached to the skeleton and allowing us action and movement at will. These are the striated muscles, the red meat we see on the butcher's slab, and they are able to contract and shorten with lightning speed when stimuli are applied to the relevant nerve; we shall come back to this point in a minute. Secondly, there are the plain or unstriped muscles, which surround the ducts of the body, constitute the greater part of the hollow organs, and form the muscular walls of the alimentary canal, and the sphincters, etc. These powerful muscles contract and relax slowly in automatic movements, and are free from voluntary control, although a yogi can reach a state where they can be controlled – but that is another story.

In relaxation it is the first group with which we are concerned, and we must be careful to dissociate the muscle from the nerve which stimulates it to action. We may compare the muscle to an electro-magnet, and its nerve to the electric wire which connects it to the mains – the brain – and from there we can go on to examine the various states in which these voluntary muscles may be found.

1. *The Latent Period of the Muscle – Incomplete Tetanus*
In their quiescent state, muscles are like soldiers on watch, uniformed and ready in barracks to rise to the attack. A weak current circulates in the conductor-wires and the electro-magnet is barely magnetized.

2. *Contraction of a Muscle*
As and when required, and in response to a message from the brain centres, a more intensive current passes through the conductor-wire activating the electro-magnet, which takes up its normal work: the muscle contracts, the arm bends, the fist clenches. The greater the effort, the larger the number of minute electro-magnetic motors set in motion thereby.

3. *Relaxation of the Muscle*
During sleep man turns away from the outside world, his needs satisfied – the Ministers for Foreign Affairs and Defence give orders for calm to be observed on every front, the soldiers take off their battle-

dress, and go on leave. In the mains the current falls, the electro-magnet is almost entirely demagnetized, out of action, the muscles soft and limp. The troops however are not all on leave–for reasons of security some detachments remain on the alert.

4. *Super-Relaxation*
The three states already described are normal and customary and occur in man as in other animals, many–even thousands–of times a day. It is however possible, through conscious and voluntary action, to disconnect more totally than in sleep those wires which lead to the various electro-magnets, thus reducing the consumption of nervous-impulses to the minimum. This is what yogic relaxation is–super-repose which in a few minutes relieves fatigue more effectively than many hours of indifferent sleep.

5. *Contraction*
There is yet another state, abnormal–yet frequent–diametrically opposed to the last, and this is the state of contraction, when the mains pour too much current into the conductor-wires, setting the electro-magnets into action quite unnecessarily, thereby wasting nervous energy as much as muscular, and leaving muscle groups in a state of perpetual contraction. This state is not normal in animals, but a great many modern city-dwellers suffer from it, alas, all too often.

How many people live with perpetually tightened jaw muscles, tense neck muscles, frowning brows, hardened shoulder muscles? There is a continuous leakage of current, a constant loss of energy, of bleeding from the nerve impulses. This output of nervous energy is waste, and its volume depends more on the number of motor-muscles brought into play than on their individual strength. Since almost as much nervous impulse is needed to contract a small face muscle as, for example, a large leg muscle, then the expenditure of energy will be in proportion both to the number of motor-nerves activated, and to the intensity of the current circulating in each of the conductor wires. A forester, for example, uses relatively little nervous energy to do a large amount of muscular work, while a public speaker uses a great deal, since he puts a large number of small muscles to work. A shorthand-typist uses more than a black-smith, which explains why silence is so valuable in husbanding that energy. Imagine what happens when you speak. An idea rises from the depths of your unconscious and forms in your mind. It must be translated at once into words supplied by your unconscious mind, in the correct grammar and syntax. Just think of the countless precise orders which have to be sent out to the muscles in order to contract and relax the vocal cords, and to vary the amount of air used – all in order to allow you to speak. Think of the countless contractions of tongue muscles, jaws, lips, face, even the hands which play their part in expression by gesticulating. Thousands of small motors each requiring their own allotment of current participate in this activity. Is it therefore so surprising that a speech lasting perhaps two hours may 'empty' a man? Very few people can speak at such length without feeling exhausted – unless they understand and practice yogic techniques for reviving the nervous system. In that case they will hold the floor effortlessly for hours on end. Therefore this justifies the practice of silence so recommended by Swami Shivananda. But the mental process of speech must be halted as well, because 'talking to oneself' is almost as tiring in terms of 'nervous current' as talking out loud. When you think in words, every part of the speech equipment except the vocal cords goes through the motions which are required for speaking aloud.

Clearly then it is not only the purely 'mechanical' outward silence that counts, but the silence from within as well. Relaxation is yoga in the pure state, since the mind controls the body entirely – disconnecting the conductor wires one by one, reducing the flow of current to the electro-magnets of the muscles throughout the body almost to nil. As yogis see it, this is the ideal exercise for the will, which is not just a hard and dictatorial power that cracks the whip but a gentle and patient wish. There is no question during relaxation of employing the 'obdurate' Western type of will. It is impossible to 'enforce' relaxation, and the mastery of mind over body is the most effective method of attaining it, without constraint and violence.

Before we examine in detail how to relax absolutely, we must first run through the postures used in relaxation, the most important of which is called 'Shavāsana' – literally the 'Corpse' posture. Is this macabre expression really so ill-chosen?

Have you never heard, when the last respects to the dead have been paid, and the funeral is over, someone saying wonderingly of the deceased: 'He is more beautiful in death than when he was alive!' He has become so because death has made him relax completely:

his features are no longer tense, and a strange beauty shines from his face – a beauty which could have been his increased tenfold while he lived, had he ever learned to relax. There can be no real beauty without relaxation; the most lovely woman is never really beautiful if she frowns; conversely a relaxed face is never ugly, for it gives out a mysterious charm.

Practise relaxation, diffuse calm, peace and harmony around you and you will become the centre of attraction! The choice of the lugubrious-sounding 'Corpse posture' reflects the Eastern attitude towards death. To us it is the end of an individual being, which is why our funerals are occasions for mourning. To the Oriental, who believes, rightly or wrongly, in reincarnation, death is a merciful incident in the evolutionary cycle, and does not carry the tragic implications which we attribute to it. In this light therefore it is not a tragedy.

Generally Shavāsana is the only relaxation posture known in the West, but in India yogis use many others for this purpose, notably when lying on the side, and excellent for sleeping. They do not advise sleeping on the back, for then the mouth falls open and leads sometimes to snoring. It is best to sleep on the left side. Why? Because, according to Western theory, the stomach is supported properly when the body is on this side, while it is misplaced on the other. The yogic explanation is different: on the left side the right-hand nostril is freed and breathing takes place through it all night. Being acutely perceptive, yogis have proved this practice to be beneficial.

Learn both these positions so as to find which gives you the maximum degree of comfort. Before we describe them, let us hear what one Western adept has to say: 'If yoga had given me nothing more than relaxation, it would have been wonderful enough.' You too will share his view once you have discovered it.

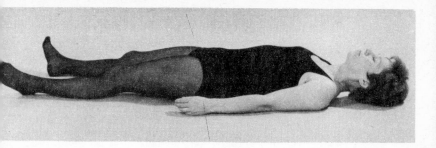

The classic position for relaxation, and the best-known posture in the West, is Shavāsana–the Corpse posture. The legs are placed slightly apart, the arms lie gently alongside the body, hands turned up or slightly inwards, fingers half-closed. The head must be laid very carefully on the floor in a position which will avoid contracting the neck muscles. Always relax on a hard surface–if necessary a cushion may be placed in the small of the back and at the nape of the neck.

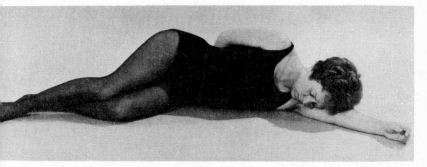

To relax on the side, lay one leg over the other, so that the knees and ankles are touching. One arm is stretched out beneath the head, the other hangs lightly over the hip. This position is not suited to prolonged exercise in relaxation.

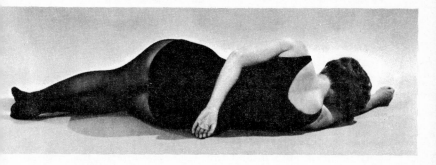

The same viewed from behind.

9. *Relaxation (continued) Its essentials*

Before sowing we must prepare the soil; before we set about practising total relaxation, we must examine the conditions preliminary to its experience.

Anyone who has mastered the art of relaxation remains relaxed in every situation–whether driving through dense traffic in a city at the rush-hour, listening to a concert, or discussing business affairs. Wherever he may be he is master of himself, relaxed, neither tense nor frowning with worry. His relaxation has become a habit independent of what is going on. But in order to attain this result, and to give it the best possible chances of success, total relaxation must be practised under the most favourable conditions. First of all and as far as possible you must get rid of any sensory stimuli and take refuge in a room where you will not be disturbed. Ensure that those around you will leave you in peace for those few minutes in the day you have put aside for practice. Draw the curtains so that the room is in half-darkness. If it has been well-aired in advance then it is as well to shut the windows to lessen noises from the street. The temperature should be comfortable, and it is also as well to cover oneself with a light warm blanket, since during relaxation the body temperature falls, and any feeling of cold will detract from success. Nothing must stand in your way, so if you are fully dressed, at least take off your belt, collar and shoes.

Now to create a suitable atmosphere for relaxation. All of us experience problems and anxieties; put them to one side while the exercises last. Tell yourself, 'Anxiety sets up tensions which prevent me from solving my problems. It is essential for me to relax before I can resolve them; this exercise is therefore the only important thing in my life at this moment.' Now think: 'I am calm and relaxed.' Look in the glass and smile. Childish? Maybe, but if it does the trick? And how can you tell unless you try? When you have set aside your worries, yawn, stretch, and rub your eyes. Pretend that you are sleepy and tired. There is no point in describing the procedure; your own instincts will tell you how. As you stretch yourself, extend and separate your fingers. If you do not know what to do next, try to imitate a cat, which always makes a regular ritual of stretching itself. First of all stretch while you are lying on your back, then roll over on to your left side, and repeat the whole operation on your right side. When you have yawned and stretched carefully you will be in a 'non-active' frame of mind, because the practice of relaxation is an exercise in 'non-activity'; although this sounds like a truism it is in fact a basic principle, often ignored. Don't tell yourself that you are going to do an exercise, but put yourself into a *laissez aller* frame of mind, letting yourself go – this is the main essential.

A test follows which allows you both to control and to practise your capacity for 'non-action'.

Stand up, feet apart, leaning the trunk forward almost at right angles to the legs. Then let the arms hang loosely in front. By turning the shoulders from left to right, swing the arms like the pendulum of a clock. Make sure that they and the hands are really swinging, without taking an active part in the movement. When the pendulum action is properly set in motion, stop the movement of the shoulders, and allow the arms to move freely from left to right under the impetus which they have acquired. The scope of the swinging action lessens quickly; let each arm come to rest gradually like the pendulum of a clock running down. Concentrate on what is happening in your arms and hands. If your hands are not completely limp and relaxed start the exercise again, having first shaken them from the wrists so that the fingers turn freely with the movement of the hands. Go on with the exercise until only the pendulum-like action is guiding the hands and arms, without any muscular intervention on your part; you can see now how they can participate in a passive manner. To control relaxation in the arms, sit on the ground, or on a chair. Let your right hand and arm hang inert, as they did when you were swinging them. Take hold of the middle or index finger of the right hand with your left, and raise the arm. If possible, ask a friend to control its relaxation, raising it by pulling on the index finger and then making it swing from left to right. You and your assistant should get the impression of dealing with a dead weight hanging from the index finger like a ham from a hook. Your assistant should now release your finger without any warning and if the arm is correctly relaxed, it will fall back inert. You will have some idea of the nature of the state your arm should be in if you lift up the arm of a sleeping child or the paw of a resting cat.

Now to experiment with the gravity which is in the whole body; in the pleasant warmth of a bath you feel relaxed and rested by the heat of the water and by the force of gravity, because in the bath you weigh practically nothing. Then pull out the plug and allow the water to run away. As your limbs emerge, you will feel yourself drawn down to the bottom of the bath and you will collapse like a puppet with no strings–feeling heavy. Learn to evoke this sensation of heaviness whenever you want to, without water, and you have reached the first stage in relaxation. Another way to achieve this is to lie in the Shavāsana posture, arms at your sides, palms turned up. Feel the way in which the earth draws every cell in your arm, every molecule and atom of it. Think of the power of the earth's attraction, and let your arm go with it. Let it lie heavily on the carpet. Try to raise it by tensing the muscles of the elbow only, and you will see how heavy it is. It will be several days before you can experience this feeling of gravity, but never mind, it will come; the main thing is to concentrate on the arm and allow it to respond to the pull of gravity. Then you can practise relaxing first the hand, finger by finger, then the palm, the wrist, the forearm, and the rest of the arm to the shoulder. Even if you do not manage to relax it entirely you must realize that you are nevertheless succeeding in a very important exercise; the localization of tension centres and of contracted muscles of which you must first be conscious before you can hope to eliminate them. And so you are not wasting your time if the exercise is not a complete success; the essential thing is to persevere. In most cases some result will be achieved and a degree of success will follow after a few days of patient trial. Each attempt will reward you with a pleasant feeling of restfulness and relaxation. The arm-relaxing exercise may be practised anywhere–should you be forced to wait about for something or other somewhere, then use the opportunity to practise relaxation, so that the apparent futility of wasted time will, instead of getting on your nerves help you to relax.

10. *Now to Deeper Relaxation*

Each day, deep down in our tissues, millions of cells die, and are replaced by others. On the other hand our nerve cells are *not* renewed. We are born with them and normally they die with us. They are the deep-seated physical foundation of what we call our 'personality'.

If we drive them too hard, if we exhaust them, then we injure and destroy them, and, since they are not replaceable, we shorten our lives. Relaxation opens the way to the inside world, to the yoga of the mind, since it is impossible to concentrate if the body is knotted with tension.

And so we aim to relax our muscles completely and to induce the most sophisticated form of hypotonia that we can.

The preceding exercises were designed to prepare you by degrees for this total relaxation which induces a deliciously light sensation – a euphoria which must be experienced to be appreciated fully. You can now take the next step while still lying flat on your back on the floor in the Shavāsana posture.

First notice your breathing: it is taking place without any intervention on your part. Concentrate your mind on the act of breathing without trying to influence it. This is more difficult than it seems at first because the mere fact that one becomes conscious of respiratory movements leads one to attempt to modify them (albeit unconsciously).

Let yourself breathe. Observe where and how you are breathing and in what rhythm. If from the top of the chest, where is the breath located? When breathing, the centre of gravity should lie in the middle of the abdomen between the navel and the sternum. While you are lying down and motionless your oxygen needs are minimal, and so the respiratory movements are also substantially lighter. The essential is to ascertain where and how you are breathing and then to allow a rhythm to establish itself, slowly, calmly and peacefully. If your breathing is encumbered, or if its rhythm is irregular, regulate it by saying to yourself: 'My breathing is becoming calm and

peaceful. My stomach is rising and falling calmly and regularly.'
Continue until you sense this inner calm, this peaceful breathing.
From that moment you will feel more relaxed. Your next task is to
influence your out breathing, slowing it down, but *not deepening
it in quality*. Let yourself exhale spontaneously, making no attempt
to force the breath further than it seems to want to go; it is enough
to slow down the exhalation to half the speed of the inspiration.
Why should it be twice as slow? Because this is the natural state.
Watch a sleeping cat and you will realize that easy exhalation
occupies twice the breathing-in period. The same applies to a
baby. Breathing and relaxation are linked together. After an
exhalation retarded in this way, stop breathing for a second or two.
During this time, *concentrate on the solar plexus*. You may reasonably
object that it is impossible to do this since you cannot feel the solar
plexus. Then simply concentrate your mind on the respiration's
centre of gravity; that is the hollow of the stomach, a little above the
navel. Now imagine that this region is being warmed by the breath
entering and leaving it. If necessary imagine you are lying in the
sun, and that it is warming this part of your body. Go on until you
feel that special sensation which comes from sunbathing on a hot
day – a kind of shiver. Now to a new stage. Concentrate effortlessly
on the right arm and hand. Relax your fingers, one by one, thumbs
included, so that there is no muscular action in the palm. If the back
of the hand is resting on the floor the fingers will be slightly flexed.

Once you have mastered the above exercise you should be able to
relax your arms and hands rapidly and completely, making them
go quite limp. You will have learnt to identify the feeling of weight,
and the next stage is to induce a feeling of warmth. No auto-
suggestion is involved! Once you can relax the muscles in a given
part of the body, the shape of the blood vessels changes; they
stretch and dilate, which in turn creates heat. Conversely when
you are tense and tightened up the spastic contraction of the
blood vessels reduces their size, and the circulation, leading to a
sensation of cold.

The blood flow in a relaxed muscle increases, and the breathing
of the cells deepens in consequence, while the body temperature rises.
When vascular spasms give you freezing hands, it is no auto-
suggestion but a proven fact.

DIAGRAM ILLUSTRATING COMPLETE RELAXATION

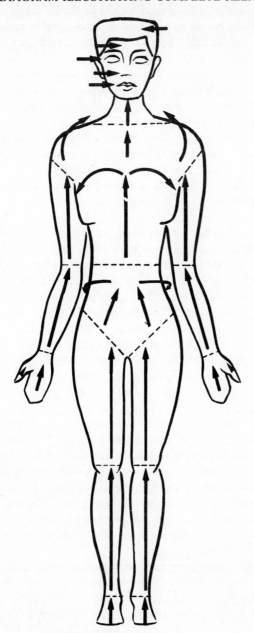

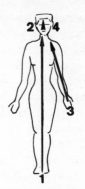

GENERAL DIRECTION
OF RELAXATION.

If you practise the exercises I have just described, then total deep relaxation is within your grasp: all you have to do is to relax every muscle in every part of your body, from feet to head, stage by stage.

But why from feet to head?

Because experiments have proved that the larger muscles are the easiest to relax, and therefore it is logical to begin with the large leg muscles at the bottom, and to work up to the face which contains the smallest muscles in the body.

During total relaxation the body must be kept absolutely motionless, for the least movement, designed for instance to control the relaxation of an arm, would re-tense the muscles, and so defer complete relaxation. There is no point in seeking to check whether you are relaxing, because for the first few minutes there is no special sensation.

Now concentrate on your body, first relaxing the feet, toes, instep, heels, and then the calves. Proceed by minute stages upwards from joint to joint, i.e. from ankle to knee; then from knee to hip, without attempting to relax the leg in a single movement. At the hip relax the abdomen, then around the waist, the muscles at the base of the spine, and then those in the stomach region. Work upwards towards the top of the chest, round the rib-cage, finally relaxing the top of the back. The next stage is to relax the neck (the throat, where the thyroid gland lies) then the face, where care must be taken to include the numerous little muscles one by one, since some of them are permanently in a state of contraction. At the face begin by relaxing the lower jaw.

You may find at this stage, that when your mouth is closed, your teeth are permanently clenched. Allow the lower jaw to fall without opening the mouth. Do not forget to relax the tongue which must lie limply inside the mouth. Then relax the muscles which surround the mouth, lips and the nostrils. Let the cheeks go limp; this will remove any expression from the face. In this way you will assume the impassive features of the oriental and your expression will be impenetrable betraying emotion only when you wish it. But we digress.

Next come the eyes, and those must be relaxed meticulously Close the lids gently over the eyeballs, without squeezing or allowing them to vibrate or flicker. Now the forehead. So many people frown unconsciously! The wrinkles caused by anxiety are seen there as well as in the nape of the neck, and in the shoulders, hence the expression 'lined with care'. Now relax the scalp. Having been over the body systematically we move on to the tips of the fingers. Relax each finger in turn, not forgetting the thumbs; stretch the palms and the wrists, work up the forearm to the elbow, then as far as the shoulders, relaxing the arm muscles as you go. After the shoulders and the shoulder-blades, relax the nape, and working over the ears, return to the cheeks, nostrils, eyes, forehead and scalp. Relaxing the face is so difficult that it is as well to practise it a second time. Having gone over the entire body from feet to head repeat the operation, and you will realize how in the meantime, certain muscles have already re-contracted. The second time round goes more quickly than the first. Should you have time—why not just make it?—run over the same tour of relaxation for a third time.

The next stage shows us how to recognize the *state of relaxation*.

Up to now you will have noticed no special sensation; you will have remained strictly motionless as was agreed, and there has been nothing to indicate whether or not you are succeeding. The first sign to assure you that all is going well is the sensation of *gravity*.

This consists in the realization that the whole body is subject to the earth's attraction. If necessary, form a mental picture of the earth as a gigantic magnet—which in fact it is—drawing your body to it. Every fibre, each cell and drop of blood, every atom of your being, is subject to this attraction. You can feel the force of gravity pulling at your feet, calves and legs. Feel them becoming heavier and heavier. Once again this is not just auto-suggestion, but an acute perception of something which, although not experienced in the normal state, is sensed when the muscles become relaxed. Feel how your trunk weighs on the carpet, irresistibly drawn down by the earth. How heavy your head is! The lower jaw and the cheeks are the regions of the face in which the force of gravity is most apparent. From your head pass on to your hands, and let them become inert and heavy. Then to the forearms and the entire length of the arms, and let the shoulders sink down. If possible run quickly through the whole operation a second and a third time to get the feeling of the force of gravity throughout the body.

Once you have reached this stage you will find you are able to sense a feeling of unbelievable relaxation, in which the body is forgotten and seems to have become insubstantial.

What is the physiological mechanism behind this feeling? During the first part of the exercise, while the muscles are being relaxed, the motor nerves are disconnected, and stop sending orders. The motor nerve cells immediately fall into a state of rest, followed rapidly by the sensory nerve cells (those which transmit sensory messages to the brain). This is what produces the extraordinary and delicious sensation of gradual detachment and lack of consciousness of the body. After a time one has the impression of floating outside one's own body, a feeling which may be disconcerting to the unprepared, but which characterizes total relaxation. With practice it is induced more and more quickly, gaining in depth meanwhile. If you do not attain this state at the first attempt you must not be surprised nor lose heart, since that is quite normal. Keep at it! It can sometimes take weeks to achieve, but meanwhile the exercise is in no way unrewarding.

By means of relaxation, the nerve cells are thoroughly invigorated: relieved for a time of the burden of directing the body's movements and of transmitting sensory messages, they derive more rest from a few minutes of relaxation than from many long hours of restless sleep. This state of 'super-rest' allows them to recuperate at maximum speed. The secret of those men renowned for their physical and mental endurance often lies in their ability to cut contact quickly and completely. Napoleon, for example would allow himself frequent intervals of several minutes' complete relaxation during the day, so that he could return to his command refreshed and alert.

This state of complete hypotonia is a point of departure. It is not the main aim; the crowning achievement is the relaxation of the psyche. Physical relaxation is a preparation for this psychical relaxation, which then produces an increased depth of physical relaxation. The state of complete bodily relaxation is the launching-pad for the discovery of a marvellous inner world, which the experienced yoga adept will finally reach: the point at which physical yoga runs into the mental. When the relaxation exercise is over, you must, slightly regretfully, make contact with the everyday world again, and recall the muscles and nerves to their normal state of vigilance. Do this by clenching the hands harder and harder, stretching, rubbing the eyes and yawning as if you had woken from deep and restorative sleep. These remarks do not apply to the relaxation which is practised before you go to sleep and which ends in slumber. One more point at this juncture. Insomniacs sometimes wish to use relaxation techniques to induce sleep without the help of drugs, and they fail, which is not surprising, because relaxation must be practised daily before it can be used as an aid to sleep. This is easy to understand: the beginner needs to put so much active thought into his relaxation, that the brain remains clear. This does not in any way hinder relaxation in the daytime, but, on the other hand, it can prevent sleep, a paradox, but a self-evident one.

LIGHTNING RELAXATION

There is not always enough time for a complete relaxation exercise requiring from fifteen to twenty minutes. We should therefore practise lightning relaxation, lying on the back, and allowing each muscle in the body to turn, as it were, into soft clay, so that we resemble a puppet whose strings have been cut. This lightning relaxation which takes only a few seconds or one or two complete breaths is practised by yogis between asanas. Emulate them, even if you cannot attain those heights of perfection, which can only be acquired gradually.

Throughout the day take any opportunity you can to fit in bouts of lightning relaxation, even when sitting down; there is no question of wasted time because you will derive such enormous benefits in the stabilization of your nerves.

11. *Self-awareness*

A yoga session is made up of:

(a) exercises to warm up the muscle-structure in preparation for the asanas. Salutation to the Sun (see p. 224) is the 'nucleus' of this 'setting in motion';
(b) self-awareness;
(c) the series of asanas enclosed in a state of total relaxation in Shavāsana.

The 'setting in motion', is done by fairly rapid movements, which induce a certain degree of cardiac and respiratory acceleration, without leading to any shortness of breath. Before initiating the series of asanas, some time will elapse until the pulse and breathing return to their normal rhythm. This time should be devoted to the period of *self-awareness*, which should be a transitional state halfway between everyday life and the asana session, representing an oasis of calm and peace within the tumult of life. During the asanas the mind controls the movements of the body. This is the essential and indeed the very foundation of yoga. But it is impossible for the mind to concentrate on the alternate contraction and relaxation of the various groups of muscles of which it can only vaguely be conscious. A civilized adult too – working almost entirely with his brain – is only obscurely conscious of his own body. So many people realize they are tense and frowning, but are unable to pinpoint exactly where the tensions lie. Many human beings breathe imperfectly and superficially, and do not even know whether they are breathing from the abdomen, the thorax, or only from the apex of the lungs.

Children, on the other hand, are still conscious of their own bodies and it is astonishing to see how easily they can achieve the nauli[1].

This exercise which is both spectacular and effective, is one of the

---

[1] Nauli: the churning abdominal movement during which the vertical recti muscles stand out isolated in the middle of the abdominal wall, giving the impression of a continuous rolling movement through alternate contraction and relaxation.

most difficult to teach, because there is nothing to 'account for' – no 'knack'. An adult will hardly ever be able to manage it with less than four or five weeks' practice – sometimes months. Yet show it to a child without explaining it in any way, and if he feels like it he will be able to isolate his recti[1] muscles after a few attempts, and what is more, without further ado, will soon be able to 'roll' them.

If he is to discipline and perfect himself, the adult must first re-establish contact with his body. This is the aim of self-awareness.

This self-awareness will be centripetal: beginning with the outside layers of consciousness, we shall penetrate more and more deeply. This entails four successive processes in awareness (a) of the skin's contacts; (b) of muscles; (c) of breathing; and (d) of one of the deep-lying organs.

(A) SENSATIONS OF CONTACT

We first turn our attention to the skin, in order to appreciate as accurately as possible the maximum number of cutaneous sensations. Lying – preferably on the back in Shavāsana – the adept systematically registers in his mind each and every cutaneous contact The sequence is the same as the one we used in relaxation (see sketch, page 57). That is to say you begin with feeling acutely conscious of the sensation of contact between your feet and the carpet, and continue by working up along the calves and thighs, covering the whole range of tactile feelings.

At the hem of your underpants you can clearly feel the different sensation: the warmth on the thigh under the pants, the contact with the material, any elastic at the waist. Work upwards over the trunk, feeling the contact of your back with the rug, the weight of your head on the floor, the hair at the nape of your neck. The sensations, for instance, apparent in the tips of your fingers resting on the floor, are very different from those in the heels. Concentrate on the feeling in each of your fingers. If you wear a ring, generally you do not notice that it is on your finger; now re-experience the feel of the metal in contact with the skin, and do the same with your bracelet or watch-strap, after which work up your arm from elbow to shoulder feeling its touch on the carpet. By this means you will have explored the entire surface of the skin. Should you be lying in the open air, then feel and notice the rays of the sun which are warming you, and the wind as it blows over you. In brief, collect as many sensory messages provided by the skin as you possibly can.

[1] These are the straight muscles in the front of the abdomen.

Educating the muscular consciousness is a large factor in culturist methods, and although the objectives of yoga are entirely different, it is essential before we can practise it to sharpen the muscular consciousness. We now therefore attempt to feel our muscle structure, first the big groups, and then, as our perception sharpens with each exercise, we shall reach a point where we can find ourselves 'sensing' individually even the small muscles.

In order to be aware of the muscles first contract them while still on your back. Try out some minute almost imperceptible movements, move your toes one after another, concentrating upon the muscles which operate them. Feel how the whole muscular mechanism moves into action under the skin. You should no longer be attending to sensations from the outside, but only to the inner ones produced by the movements you are making. Next move your whole foot. To do this you are forced to contract the calves. Concentrate on the structure of their muscles; then contract the buttocks and the thighs. Feel the muscular masses as they come to life beneath your skin. Now the abdomen: contract the muscles in front, then at the sides, then round the waist, and in the small of your back. Go over the trunk and move any muscle you can identify, including the pectorals and the muscles in the upper region of the back. The neck should be included in this organized exploration.

Now to the face. You will find plenty of sensation in the great number of small and very mobile muscles there.

Begin by moving the jaws, slowly from left to right, without grinding the teeth. Take note of all the muscles brought into play thereby. Move the tongue, the lips, smile. Then move the nostrils, smile broadly, and feel how the cheek muscles take part in the movement. Roll your eyes, beneath your closed eyelids, squeeze, then open the eyelids, frown and relax the forehead, raise and lower the eyebrows feeling the muscles contracting under the scalp.

Next, move each finger separately beginning at the tip, clench the fists, and watch the results in the muscles of the forearm. Tense the shoulders, the biceps, and all the muscles which lie around the humerus.

There is no limit to the number of muscles you can become aware of: the more you can identify, the more successful the exercise will prove.

For the moment we shall leave the subject of muscular activity in order to dwell on the breathing, which is normally unconscious. Since, however self-awareness has already been dealt with (see p. 19) we shall not enlarge on it here.

Briefly we should remember that the main requirement is to observe our breathing. Try to be aware of how it works *without* any direct intervention on your part: do not breathe–just allow your breathing to take place, observing where and how, no more.

Having consciously listened to this for a while, slow down the process of exhalation, which should last twice as long as inspiration. After five to ten such respirations, we are ready to pass on to the final stage of the exercise: the act of becoming consciously aware of an individual organ.

Yogis reach a point where they are able to observe and control their internal organs: heart, stomach, liver, spleen, intestines and so on.

We shall not be so ambitious, because the practice is not devoid of danger when done without supervision from a qualified instructor. On the other hand it is desirable, for reasons we shall explain later, to be conscious of the heart. When holding the breath with the lungs full of air, certain precautions must be taken, but there is no danger when they are emptied. Hold the breath with emptied lungs for a few seconds (as you progress you will be able to increase the time substantially). While doing so, focus your mind on the epigastric region between the navel and the sternum (breast bone). You will become conscious of your heartbeat, sometimes even at your first attempt.

You may ask whether it is advisable to concentrate on your heartbeats. Let me explain: your health depends above all upon the sympathetic nervous system, which regulates all automatic functions of the body; the heartbeats, the workings and activities of the lungs, stomach, and alimentary canal, as well as the accessory glands, the heart-regulating mechanism and so on. In fact the whole internal structure of the organism. All this activity is ruled by the controlling action of the ortho-sympathetic nervous and the pneumogastric or vagus systems. The pneumogastric nerve, as its name implies, activates the lungs, heart and stomach, and loses itself within the complex network of the solar plexus.

As soon as concentration is focused on the breathing, especially when this is held, your conscious self imposes its will on your automatic self, and takes over. Therefore, while you are holding your breath, your conscious mind takes possession of the automatic movements at the medulla oblongata – the vital organ situated at the junction of the spinal cord with the brain. While you concentrate on the heartbeat, your awareness slowly breaks through to encompass the pneumogastric nerve leading to the heart, and now you are breaking new ground. This is how yogis came to be aware of the automatic functions, a matter of mere academic interest to ourselves, since we have decided not to emulate them. Nevertheless it is very much worth while to observe your heartbeats, and to hold your breath; to think of that part of the *self* which you normally ignore, and which maintains the temperature of your body, digests your food, etc., with very little fuss. You are to make friends with this unseen and unknown part of your Self!

Now awareness has been fully achieved. It is clearly impossible to arrive at this sort of complete self-awareness in two or three minutes, which is the transition period laid down between the preparatory stages and the postures.

Yet with practice you will be able to cut it down to three minutes, quickly passing through the various stages. Before your yoga session, make do with a 'lightning' exercise in self-awareness. A long one may be carried out in bed on awakening, or in the evening. Although the position may be the same as that taken up for relaxation, you must not confuse the two exercises, which are almost directly opposed; whereas in muscular relaxation you 'forget' the body, here you are attempting to be as completely conscious of it as you can.

12. *The Secret of a Supple Body*

I nearly wrote 'the secret of youth', because one of the fundamental differences between a young body and an ageing frame lies in the contrast between the flexibility of the one and the stiffness of the other. In other words *suppleness of youth*.

Yoga adepts remain extraordinarily, superlatively supple until advanced age. In the ashrams of India the 'seniors' are often more supple than the younger inmates.

The secret of this suppleness imparted by Hatha-yoga is quite simple: relaxed muscles lengthen as a result of slow and progressive traction. To stretch muscles after relaxing them is one of the essential characteristics of the asanas. That is why this form of exercise produces flexibility in the body more thoroughly and quickly than gymnastics, which are designed to develop the muscular structure of the body through repeated contractions of the voluntary muscles. A sporting activity is judged by the number of muscles it seeks to strengthen. Although the present tendency in the West is to introduce phases of rapid relaxation between the movements, this relaxation differs fundamentally from that produced by yogic asanas.

Let us go over something of what we have learnt about the physiology of the voluntary (striated) muscles.

They are normally to be found in three differing states:

(a) *In contraction*. This is the 'useful' period of activity during which the muscle, by shortening itself, acts upon the skeleton and supplies the mechanism whereby movement can take place. It is almost the sole basis of gymnastic exercise and sport.

(b) *In a state of tone*. This is the normal state for the 'awakened' muscle – latent but nevertheless prepared to contract as soon as some order reaches it through an impulse of the nerve.

(c) *When relaxed*. Here the muscle is 'at rest'. It is in this state during sleep and while yogic relaxation is being practised. These three states are normal, general and familiar[1].

To these another must be added – exceptional in everyday life – the *stretched* muscle.

This state is unusual and completely different from the other three, in that the muscle cannot stretch itself, but must be stretched through an exterior action. Since stretching is used systematically in each of the asanas, it is essential to grasp the nature of this muscular attribute so that you can carry out the postures correctly, and understand their effect better.

The elasticity of muscle is quite different from that of rubber, which can be stretched until it tears. Muscle is easily stretched and can be extended within 'normal limits of elasticity'. When these limits are reached, the muscle may then be lengthened further, but only *slowly*. The more relaxed it is the more amenable to stretching. A sharp pull on a muscle which is not relaxed may even injure it. Slow continuous and progressive traction on a relaxed muscle is completely safe: what is more it induces a series of good effects, the first of which is that blood, especially when venous, is squeezed out. The circulation of venous blood does not depend on cardiac impulses, but on the alternate contraction and relaxation of the muscles, which, by compressing the veins, expel the blood in the direction of the heart. But it is only by the action of stretching that the muscle can be properly emptied. As soon as the activity ceases the muscle returns to its normal size and 'breathes in' fresh blood which serves to bathe, cleanse and nourish it.

Furthermore, and this explains why asanas induce greater flexibility faster than any other method, each stretching extends the normal elasticity limit of the muscle so that the body becomes progressively more and more supple.

CONCLUSIONS: A GUIDE TO PRACTICE
Since, during each asana, certain groups of muscles are stretched, you should concentrate carefully on these *before* and *during* the traction which must be *slow* and *progressive*. The Forward Bend (Paschimottānāsana), for instance, stretches the muscles of the back,

[1] In this chapter we shall not consider this state of rest as an exercise in relaxation, but rather as an integral part of each asana.

and you will soon find these have reached their limit. However if you wait a few moments relaxed in this position, you will realize that by gradually pulling on the arms you will gain a few centimetres. This is why repeated, jerky movements are not permitted in yoga: they prevent muscular relaxation, an essential preliminary to any stretching movement.

This muscular relaxation outside sleep is a voluntary and there-fore conscious act which calls for your undivided concentration on the asanas. The more completely you *live* them, the more attentive and concentrated you will be, and therefore the more completely relaxed and better able to stretch your muscles. You will become supple quickly and painlessly. This mental concentration is an excellent exercise in the discipline of the mind and is a preparation for Rāja-yoga. Some adepts find it helps to practise with their eyes *closed*. It is also necessary to relax at great speed, and as thoroughly as possible before and between each posture, which is why almost all asanas begin from a recumbent position. Before practice, ensure that you are relaxed and then proceed, using the smallest possible number of muscles and limiting their contractions to a strict mini-mum. Continue normal breathing (except where otherwise indicated), while you are in the posture. In the final posture take particular care to relax those muscles which the asana directly affects. Carry out the traction slowly and in a continuous movement, and then return to the floor. Breathe deeply and completely and relax once more. While you are resting on the floor, the blood *flows in great quantity* into the muscles which have been stretched. This relaxation is one of the absolutely essential stages, and you should not rush from one posture to the next: yoga does not countenance haste! Do not begin the next asana until the breathing and heartbeats have returned to normal. This relaxation may be cut short between two postures of the same kind, which are devised to bend the body in the same direction; for instance, between the Cobra posture, the Locust and the Bow, it is not necessary to rest for as long as between the Bow and the Forward Bend.

These fundamentals can lead on to unlimited improvements.

Remember that proper preparation before an asana can make your work much easier, because muscles which have first been warmed up will stretch with greater ease.

13. *Concentration during Asanas*

Although it is possible to benefit from Western methods of physical exercise done without regard to mental attitude or to concentration of the mind, yet the latter, when used in conjunction with relaxation, is indispensable to the study of yoga as well as to the asanas.

But how to concentrate and on what? Throughout this book we shall always indicate where to concentrate during each asana, but you should also be aware of the general rules of concentration: the ancient treatises refer to the points on which the attention must focus, but they were formulated for accomplished experts, and concentration on these lines is neither possible–nor even desirable– until the technique of the asanas has been perfected. The fact that the beginner should concentrate on different aspects than the expert is too often ignored or forgotten.

A. DURING THE ACTIVE OR DYNAMIC STAGE
The focus for concentration varies according to whether the active or static stage of the asana is being practised–and also according to the degree of progress reached by the student.

1. *Concentration upon Correct Method*
The beginner should first concentrate upon acquiring the *correct technique,* until he reaches the stage when he knows it by heart and can carry out the movement with the almost automatic ease with which he controls his motor car.

2. *Concentrating on Relaxation*
This first stage can be covered in a few days or weeks at the most, after which we move on to concentrating on performing the asana with as much economy as possible, that is to say in using the minimum number of muscles, with the least amount of contractions, at

the same time ascertaining that the other groups of muscles remain relaxed.

This second stage, often more prolonged than the first, is essential and must not be by-passed. Do not forget to relax the face, especially the mouth and tongue. During this stage, the beginner will find it helps to keep a picture in the mind: in the Plough posture, for example, he should try to imagine that his feet have become very light, so that when he has relaxed and tries to raise them, contracting only the abdominal region, he will be surprised at the ease with which they will rise up.

3. *Concentration upon Breathing*

Once the adept is able to manage the movement in a relaxed and semi-automatic manner, then he must find out whether he is breathing normally and smoothly (unless otherwise advised) throughout the movement. Only very advanced experts can deviate from this rule if told to do so by their *guru*. Normal breathing must be continued, for if it is stopped, the diaphragm is blocked and becomes congested. When a beginner raises the legs while lying flat on his back he tends to hold his breath, which is at once noticeable–his face becomes crimson.

4. *Concentrating on a Consistently Smooth Performance*

And now to the final stage. If the true yogic method of performance is to be used in an asana (still taking the Plough posture as an example), the adept raises his legs, the toes travel at a consistently slow rate until they touch the ground behind his head, and likewise on the return. The yogi cannot accept either a jerky, hasty, or slowing-down movement, and his continuous and smooth performance marks him out from the beginner. The casual spectator watching the performance of asanas which are clearly a pleasure to execute, receives an impression of calm strength, resembling that of a great river running slowly but surely towards the sea. Asanas practised in this way lead automatically to concentration: since different groups of muscles are engaged in succession, the co-ordination needed to maintain the movement at a strictly consistent rate completely engrosses the mind.

1. *Concentrating on Remaining Motionless and Relaxed*

The beginner should concentrate on remaining absolutely still–a condition which, combined with relaxation, is the first essential of the static part of the exercise (except where contrary instructions are given). Breathing carries on normally, and can in fact increase during the motionless phase.

The expert keeps a perpetual check on muscular relaxation. In the Plough posture, for example, everything relaxes: the face, arms, hands, feet, calves, thighs and especially the muscles which are being stretched, for example those in the back. This lengthening process empties them of blood, like a sponge being squeezed, and on returning to their normal state after the posture they take up eagerly a fresh supply of blood. This stretching is the secret of suppleness in Hatha-yoga, and returns the muscles to their normal length; so many Westerners are unable to sit on the ground with their legs stretched out in front of them!

Muscles of normal length permit the body to take up a comfortable position whatever the circumstances. If those of the spine are shortened through lack of use (and this is true of almost 99 per cent of human beings in the civilized state) the spine is rigid and any slightly brusque movement, even the least violent, may result in an accidental displacement of one of the vertebrae, requiring treatment from an orthopaedic surgeon or an osteopath.

Provided the muscles are supple and of normal length, any movements may be made, since the vertebrae move freely and replace themselves properly. If the spine is rigid, the slightest fall, the slightest car accident, may have tragic consequences, but if the muscle structure is supple and strong, it can put up with shocks which would break an ordinary spine in two.

There is at least one case where a yoga expert owed her life to this suppleness. When her own small car was cannoned into by a powerful American car her door flew open, throwing her more than thirty feet to land on the pavement like a broken doll. She astonished the doctors by emerging with a slight back injury and with her cervical ligaments a little damaged!

2. *Concentration on the Strategic Point of the Asana*

When the adept can remain still and relaxed, breathing normally, he is able to concentrate on the asana's strategic point of action. *This is the intent which is written into the old manuscripts:* we can now see how much preparation we shall need before we can attain it! Each asana (and here lies one of the essential differences between yoga and every other method of physical education), produces easily assessed effects upon some part of the body: the thyroid region, for instance, is affected by the Sarvāngāsana posture, the solar plexus by the Bow posture, and so on. This is the point on which the adept will concentrate.

From then on the asana is true to Alain Daniélou's definition – the best we have yet found – that an asana represents a position in which one can keep still for a long time without effort.

These rules allow you to determine at whatever stage you have reached in your study of yoga, where and how you are to concentrate your mind.

It is interesting to see that an adept may be mastering different degrees of the various asanas, that is to say, when learning a new one he is a beginner, while for those which he has learnt thoroughly he may already have reached the most advanced stage.

14. *In What Order Should We Practise the Postures?*

Yoga has reaped the harvest of thousands of years' experience, and nothing is left to chance–the sequence of asanas is subject to the most precise ruling. Within a series each posture falls into place, completing or accentuating the previous one, preparing for the next one or acting as a counter-posture to balance another.

Among the various series of asanas you should choose one and persevere with it since, in the long-term, the organism accustoms itself–conditions itself in the Pavlovian sense of the word–and by preparing itself reacts the better.

We have chosen as an example the series which was taught at Rishikesh in the ashram of Swami Shivananda. It only takes about half-an-hour, which is well within our scope, while the series of Swami Dhirendra Bramachari of Delhi, which is far more complete and lasts for about three hours including its preliminaries, is not practicable in the West.

The following describes the 'Rishikesh' series:

SESSION OF ASANAS

CANDLE SARVĀNGĀSANA		1 MIN.
PLOUGH HALĀSANA		2 MIN. INCLUDING THE DYNAMIC STAGE
FISH MATSYĀSANA		1 MIN.
FORWARD BEND PASHCHIMOTTĀNĀSANA		2 MIN. INCLUDING THE DYNAMIC STAGE
COBRA BHUJAṄGĀSANA		1 MIN. INCLUDING THE DYNAMIC STAGE
LOCUST SHALABHĀSANA		1 MIN. INCLUDING THE HALF LOCUST
BOW DHANURĀSANA		$\frac{1}{2}$ MIN.
SPINAL TWIST ARDHA-MATSYENDRĀSANA		1 MIN.
HEADSTAND SHĪRSĀSANA		1 to 10 MINS. OR MORE.
UDDIYANA AND/OR NAULI		1 MIN. or 2 MINS.
BREATHING		3 MINS.
SHAVĀSANA RELAXATION		3 MINS.

In India no beginner thinks of questioning the instructions of a Master – whose authority is so great, his personality so transcendent, that the disciple would no more question his *guru* than a schoolboy would contradict the conclusions of one of Einstein's equations. In any case, the Master himself believes that long explanations are superfluous, and allows the adept to discover for himself how well-founded the instructions are. But, in the West, our rationalist mind demands to know the why and wherefore of yogic exercises; a legitimate desire, and one which, if it were not present, would have to be instilled, because the learner who is on his own must know the rules so that he can avoid the pitfalls.

We shall therefore analyse the 'Rishikesh series' and, while doing so, we shall learn to appreciate the intuitive genius of the Rishis of former days.

SARVĀNGĀSANA
The 'Candle' Shoulder Stand

The first asana in the series is an inverted posture, chosen for its considerable and immediate effect on the circulation of the blood and for the very small amount of muscular effort required to perform it. The force of gravity speeds up the rate of the circulation of any stagnating venous blood, which then returns to the heart by gravitational force instead of being forced to run counter to it. Sarvāngāsana gets rid of any stoppage in the veins of the legs and the abdominal organs. All inverted postures powerfully activate the circulation with almost no muscular effort. That is why some Masters recommend Shīrsāsana, the Head-stand, but we shall use Sarvāngāsana (the Candle) which is within reach of everyone, and which includes the thyroid region, stretches the nape of the neck, and liberates the nervous network of the cervical region, the essential crossroads in our bodies.

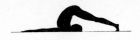

HALĀSANA
The Plough

Forward Bending
This posture, by increasing the compression of the neck, cleanses the thyroid and stretches the cervical regions (the neck and nape). It therefore increases the effects of the previous posture (Sarvāngāsana). The forward bending stretches the spinal column and the stomach is massaged. Because the thoracic cage is compressed and the rib-cage blocked, breathing is done from the stomach.

MATSYĀSANA
The Fish

Counter-posture
Matsyāsana forms a counter-position for the two preceding exercises. In other words the neck which has been compressed for a considerable time is set free.

In the inverse position, the cervicals are squeezed instead of stretched. The thorax opens widely which has a good effect upon thoracic breathing. The stomach is stretched, the back hollowed in the opposite way to the Plough, and the breathing is chiefly thoracic and clavicular.

PASCHIMOTTĀNĀSANA
The Forward Bend (sitting)

Paschimottānāsana bends the spinal column forward without compressing or pulling out the nape or the neck itself. The curve reaches in particular to the bottom part of the back which is why this asana *completes* the Plough posture. This time *the stomach* is compressed whereas in the previous posture it was stretched.

77

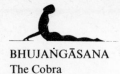

BHUJAṄGĀSANA
The Cobra

The First of a Series of Three Backward Bends
During the dynamic phase the stomach is *compressed;* during the static phase it is *stretched.*

The spinal column is bent backwards in the opposite manner to the Plough and the Forward Bend. In the Cobra the dorsal muscles, which in both the preceding postures were stretched and emptied of their blood like a squeezed sponge are about to contract; and it is possible to see how these contractions induce a great quantity of fresh blood in the back.

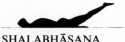

SHALABHĀSANA
The Locust

Shalabhāsana comes after the Cobra and complements it. The dynamic stage of the Cobra concerns the top of the back, from the neck to the waist, while in the Locust it is the muscular structure below the belt which contracts forcibly in order to raise the legs.

DHANURĀSANA
The Bow

Backward Bending
The Bow posture which raises the bust and the bottom of the back together, combines both Cobra and Locust, complementary asanas which have prepared the dorsal muscles and the spinal column to stand up to the accentuated curve required in the Bow, which therefore comes logically after these postures.

78

ARDHA-MATSYENDRĀSANA
The Spinal Twist

The successive bending both forwards and backwards, elaborated and repeated, induces a special sensation in the muscles, intensifying the curvature, which Ardha-Matsyendrāsana immediately corrects because it twists the spinal column in both directions. This is why the posture is placed after all the bending ones.

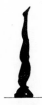

SHĪRSĀSANA
The Head-stand

The series ends with Shīrsāsana, the queen of the asanas. Some Masters place it at the beginning; however, since our series starts with Sarvāngāsana, it is contained between two inverted postures, which is very favourable.

AFTER THE ASANAS
The mudras and bandhas (movements and contractions) are done after the asanas. We shall practise Uḍḍiyāna Bandha (the abdominal squeeze), followed by some complete breaths and/or one or other of the more advanced breathing exercises.

Relaxation, even if brief, ends the session and constitutes an excellent change-over from yoga to everyday life.

HOW TO COMPLETE OR MODIFY THIS SERIES
During the Rishikesh series, the postures are completed and mutually reinforced, while if they are practised on the spur of the moment,

in no logical order they may neutralize each other or even fail to produce positive results. Research has shown how carefully they are constructed. If you wish to integrate or to substitute other postures, there is a very simple principle which will help you to avoid mistakes. Quite simply – any bend made in a forwards direction may be replaced by another in the same category. Any variation in a posture should come before or after the principal one, so long as it does not merely replace it. In this way, the structure of the series will remain unchanged and correct.

15. *Asanas*

Although asanas or yogic postures form only *one* aspect of yoga, for the Westerner leading a sedentary life they represent the main part of his practice, and they bring him tangible and quick results, while preparing him for other forms of yoga.

While Swedish gymnastics and sports which are based on external action, develop the muscles, asanas work in depth in our interior being, partly on the physical plane (viscera, endocrine glands, brain, voluntary and involuntary nervous systems), and also on the mental level, where they produce the sort of calm and serenity which may be the key to energy and happiness. The suppleness they create is unequalled (see 'The Secret of Suppleness,' p. 67);–and, with this amazing endurance there is no fatigue or nervousness. What is more, they are in their own right first-class exercises in concentration (see 'Where to concentrate during the asanas' p. 70).

But before we begin to study the more classical and the most effective postures, which anyone can achieve, we must first clarify the conditions to be observed before we practise them.

These are:

EXTERIOR FACTORS

The Time:
The best time to undertake a session of asanas is in the morning after washing and cleaning your teeth, etc; it will put you in top form for the rest of the day! If you cannot fit a morning practice into your timetable, you may work in the evening either before your meal or before going to bed, or perhaps you could even work in a second session! It is easier to make a success of it in the evening than in the morning, because the long time spent lying still overnight means that you are less supple when you wake than you are in the evening. Yet a morning practice does not detract from the asanas' good effects!

The Place:
This, if possible, should be out of doors. Ideally, asanas should be practiced at sunrise on the beach, beside a lake or on a river bank. But otherwise a garden or terrace will serve, and if neither is practicable then you can do them in a well-aired and heated room. *Never work anywhere where the air is vitiated.*

What to Wear:
As little as decency and the temperature permit. In the summer, yoga, fresh air and light may all be enjoyed together. In winter, if it is cold in the room where you are practising, then do not hesitate to cover up well (outdoor sports or 'training' clothes). Do not wear tightly-fitting garments which will hinder your circulation.

Requirements:
A rug or folded blanket (not too thick) is all you need.

PHYSICAL CONDITIONS

Fasting
This is one more reason for choosing the morning for the session! Failing this, wait four or five hours after a large meal, and two hours after a lighter one. This applies to the asanas which can upset the digestion, (the relaxation exercises and complete yogic breathing will not affect it). Empty the bladder and, if possible, the bowels before beginning.

Practise every day in the same place and at the same time, unless some major event prevents you. In this way you will 'condition' your organism to react more and more satisfactorily to the asanas. Remember Pavlov's experiments, whereby a dog was fed to the sound of a bell ringing at a certain hour. After a time, the ringing and the meal were so closely associated in the animal's brain that, even when food failed to appear, the ringing still set the salivary glands and the gastric secretions to work and these became 'conditioned reflexes'. This is the process you are consciously creating in yourself. If you are very tired, do not begin with the asanas. Devote the first minutes to yogic breathing and relaxation, then practise the postures. Women should refrain from asanas during the first few days of menstruation, and should stop them altogether from the fifth month of pregnancy onwards.

Bathing
Do not take a very hot nor a very cold bath immediately after the asanas, because this would draw the blood away to the peripheral regions of the body. During the first thirty minutes after a session, the organism continues to circulate a large amount of blood that has been accumulated in the deep-lying organs, and a very hot or very cold bath would neutralize this effect. Wait moreover, for at least half an hour before undertaking any violent exericise. A warm shower (about blood heat) on the other hand, may follow these sessions, because the temperature will not be sufficient to influence the circulation of the blood. There is nothing to prevent you from eating a meal directly after a session.

GENERAL CONDITIONS

Chapter 2 defined the spirit of yoga. After the session, the expert pauses for a while in order to achieve a state of mind in which he is able to think of the body as a sacred thing, even in its most ordinary functions.

Asanas must be correctly practised, with respect for rules which are the heritage of thousands of years' experience, handed down without a break through generations of yogis. Hatha-yoga does not admit any haste and the Western practitioner should put aside any question of precipitate action. Do not let us be hurried in our search for perfection!

Regular and daily practice will be rewarded by success: a little at a time, but each and every day. You are on the right road if, after doing the asanas you feel full of vigour and vitality. Yoga should bring you joy if not pleasure.

You are on the wrong road if you feel 'empty', or if you are really in pain after your session. You may however, at the outset find that you have slight stiffness because muscles which have hitherto been inactive for years, are now working again. Go on practising; a very few days later, the stiffness will disappear for ever!

1. Asanas are not forced exercise; they work of their own volition, not by the application of violence.

2. The slow pace of the movements is essential to the effectiveness of yoga.

3. Hold the posture for the prescribed length of time.

4. Do not tense any muscles which are not essential to maintaining the asana; relax all the others.

5. Concentrate on the regions of the body assigned to each asana.

6. The return to the starting position should also be done very slowly.

7. Between two postures, rest for a few seconds relaxing the greatest possible number of muscles, including those of the face.

8. If you are short of time, reduce the number of asanas but never quicken the pace of practice.

9. Always practise the asanas in the same order.

10. Always end your session with Shavāsana for at least one minute.

CHART ILLUSTRATING SUGGESTED PROGRESS FOR BEGINNERS

	1st stage	2nd stage	3rd stage	4th stage	5th stage	6th stage	7th stage	8th stage*
Breathing								
Self-awareness								
Salutation to the Sun			1/2/3	10/11 12	1/2/3 10/11 12	1/2/3 4/5/6	1/2/3 4/5/6 7/8/9	COMP.
Sarvāngāsana (Candle)								
Halāsana (Plough)								
Pashchimottānāsana (Forward Bend)								
Bhujangāsana (Cobra)								
Matsyāsana (Fish)								
Shalabhāsana (Locust)								
Camel								
Dhanurāsana (Bow)								
Ardha-Matsyendrāsana	SIMP.	SIMP.	SIMP.	SIMP.	COMP.	COMP.		
Kapālāsana								
Shīrṣāsana								
Uḍḍiyāna Bandha								
Relaxation								
Total time taken	15′	20′	20′	25′	25′	30′	35′	40′

It is not possible to lay down any fixed plan for beginners which will suit everyone without exception. In yoga everything is individual and personal. Practical experience in the East has, however, allowed us to choose a scale of increasing difficulty in the practice of the postures. This has led us to lay down various degrees for this training. It is a good principle to know each posture to some extent before passing on to the next. This training may take from two months to two years, according to the individual. No specific time has been laid down for the duration of each exercise, and we have left it to the individual to appoint his time as he is able, taking into account the rules laid down for the technical part of each exercise.

IMPORTANT!

The asanas described in the following pages are placed in the normal order for your session.

It could be, however, that one or other asana is not within your scope when you start. Do not linger over it. First practise the easiest in the order laid down. As and when you become more supple set yourself to practise the more difficult postures, but do not 'force' them. In yoga deliberate slowness is the secret of rapid progress! You will very soon be able to carry out with ease the asanas which eluded you in the beginning. The only condition required is respect for the correct method.

Thoroughly instil into yourself the idea that the effectiveness of an asana does not depend solely on technique, but also upon the mental concentration which goes with it.

16. *Sarvāngāsana*

'Sarva' in Sanskrit means 'all', and 'anga' means members or parts; the word therefore, is not difficult to translate. And yet some authors interpret it as 'a posture for every part of the body'. This seems reasonable, since it is a posture which acts upon the whole body by stimulating the thyroid gland; but many other asanas, especially the headstand, have a similar action. Why did the yogis choose Sarvāngāsana? As the Frenchman, Alain Daniélou affirms, Sarvāng-āsana is the ellipse of 'sarva–anga uttana–asana' (which means literally 'the posture of all the raised members'), (see photograph), which differentiates it from all the others. The English expression 'pan-physical posture', rather than the 'topsy-turvy' or any other would serve, were it permissible, but on the whole, it is easier to stick to the Sanskrit term–Sarvāngāsana.

GENERAL OBSERVATIONS

The essential part of this asana lies in the inverted body position and the stretching of the nape of the neck, with stimulation to the thyroid gland achieved through the pressure of the chin against the sternum. When we come to study Shīrṣāsana, the head-stand, we shall give a detailed description of the beneficial effects of inverting the body, but having already described Sarvāngāsana, it is worth calling brief attention to its esoteric aspect. Orientals (yogis included) acknowledge the existence of positive and negative currents (the 'Yin' and 'Yang' of the Chinese) and state that a flow of cosmic energy descends from the sky to the earth; which is why, when man is in the upright position, these currents run over him from top to toe. In inverted positions this current acts in the opposite way, and this tends to have a stabilizing effect on a human being, the only member of all creation to hold himself vertically, and the only one throughout whose body length these cosmic radiations pass in this way. This also explains the importance which yogis ascribe to purposely maintaining the spinal column in a straight line and vertical during the prānayama and meditation.

What ought we to think of these 'currents'? What does Western science have to say? Any doctor or meteorologist knows that the surface of the earth holds a negative charge, while the upper atmosphere is positive. The lower atmosphere in which we live is therefore contained in an electrostatic field, with a general downward flow which may build up to a potential of between 100 to 150 volts or more per metre.

And again, if we take the phenomena of life with special reference to those relating to nervous and cerebral activity, which have electric properties containing electrolytes, which are the real bases of life in the cells, we conclude that this current exercises considerable influence on every phenomenon in our lives.

Until now, apart from Professor Fred Vlès of the Faculty of Medicine at Strasburg, and Director of the Institute of Biological Physics,[1] as well as the Russian scientist, Tshijewski, this relationship between electricity and life has never given rise to speculation or research in the West. And yet Dr J. Belot wrote: 'When we look at life in the light of biophysics, we can see that electric phenomena are at the basis of all cellular life, and we conclude that the outcome of everything is an electric charge'.

This more than justifies the esoteric interpretation of the effects of inverted postures. The great Rishis of ancient India lit upon these subtle phenomena and their theories, which have stood for thousands of years, are now in process of being confirmed by the discoveries in modern science.

Let us recall the statement made by Yesudian: 'This posture is of such great benefit to the entire organism that everyone should practise it several times daily. Its extraordinary wholesome effect is partially due to the fact that in it we receive opposite currents. It is well known that the earth gives out negative currents while we receive positive currents from universal space. In our normal upright posture, we thus receive negative currents through our feet and positive ones through our heads. In inverted body postures (*three of which follow:* Sarvāngāsana, Shīrṣāsana and Viparīta Karani Mudrā), the effect is the opposite. The fact that the entire organism is upside-down is the cause of their great therapeutic value'.

What we can say is that Sarvāngāsana produces almost all the effects of the head-stand, without being so hard to achieve.

[1] 'The biological conditions created by the electrical properties present in the lower atmosphere'. Paris, Hermann and Co.

The asana itself is easy enough. In the final attitude, the body rests upon the shoulders and the nape of the neck – which accounts for the posture's English name – 'shoulder-stand'.

Starting position. This is identical to that of the Plough posture (Halāsana) i.e. lying flat on the back (see page 108).

First phase: Bring the legs up to the vertical position. Bring the feet up together without stretching the muscles, but with the small of the back to the floor in order not to put undue strain on the fifth lumbar vertebra and its disc. If the back is quite flat on the ground, there is no danger. If the back is very hollow the knees should be bent before the feet are raised; if the small of the back still fails to touch the ground, a soft folded towel may be placed in the hollow of the back. By contracting the abdomen, raise the legs very slowly, keeping the calves and thighs relaxed and taking care not to point the toes, which would contract the calf muscles.

The upward movement must be slow and constant. The face and arms are relaxed. Breathe calmly and evenly; do not hold the breath.

Intermediate Pauses

It is a good thing to interrupt the exercise by stopping to carry out between one and five respirations when the legs have been raised to an angle of 30°, and again at 60°.

Raising the Legs to the Vertical Position

As opposed to the Plough in which the thighs are drawn in toward the abdomen and then the chest, finally bringing the feet to rest on the ground, in Sarvāngāsana the feet are raised as high as possible through contraction of the stomach muscles, and by supporting the body with the hands and forearms on the ground. The legs, followed by the trunk, rise ever higher in order to make the body vertical so that it rests on the shoulders and the nape of the neck. The feet and knees are kept together. In the final attitude the hands push up and support the back, elbows touching the carpet, the forearms propping up the body so as to keep it vertical. The sternum rises to rest against the chin, and the nape is flat to the floor.

The dynamic stage which is little known in the West, begins when the body has reached the vertical. Each leg is slowly and alternately lowered to the floor, resolving in a half-Plough position. The leg is lowered by means of its own weight, without stiffening, the muscles as relaxed as possible. Should the toes touch the floor behind your head, you have reached perfection, but otherwise you will have to be patient – they will soon do so with no effort on your part!

Now bring up the leg to join the other one which has meanwhile remained upright and motionless. Repeat the procedure with the other leg and go through the operation a second time. Then let the feet (still together) return to the floor with the toes touching the carpet: for a brief moment you will have been in the Plough posture; without pausing bring the legs slowly back to the vertical. This ends the dynamic stage and prepares the adept for the Plough which succeeds Sarvāngāsana.

Caution
Avoid any scissor-like movement with the legs!

STATIC STAGE
The immobilisation of the body in the vertical position with the whole weight on the nape, the back of the head and shoulders, is the static stage of the asana. While it is in progress relax as many muscles as possible, from the feet to the head. Breathe freely.

Returning to the Ground
This is achieved in the opposite direction to that used in taking up the position – with or without pauses at 60° and 30°. To do this, remove the supporting hands and lower the legs a little. Slowly return, controlling each stage of the movement: allow the head to remain on the ground until the end. The spinal column should uncoil progressively onto the carpet from nape to sacrum.

BREATHING
You should continue to *breathe normally* throughout. During the static phase, this will be done almost automatically from the diaphragm.

While assuming the posture, and during the dynamic stage, when the asana position is being taken up, concentrate upon moving steadily throughout each stage, and on relaxing the muscles. Watch your breathing which must remain normal and continuous.

During the Static Stage

Concentrate on remaining motionless, on your relaxation and breathing, and when these three states are achieved together, concentrate on the throat where the thyroid gland lies.

VERY IMPORTANT

The posture's inverted position is largely responsible for its beneficial effects, which bring a rush of blood to the head, and lead to compression of the throat; it is therefore very important that the chin should touch the sternum.

MISTAKES

—Do not assume the posture when the back is hollowed and unsupported. This throws the body out of alignment and sets up immense pressure on the fifth lumbar vertebra.

—Do not work in jerks.

—Do not kick off to reach the vertical position: if you find this impossible, then use a wall to help you, and place the hands under the buttocks, or, alternatively, approach the posture by way of a half-Sarvāngāsana (see 'For Beginners' overleaf).

(The chin should rest on the chest; the nape of the neck should be laid flat on the floor in the final position; failing to do so would greatly detract from the beneficial effects of the exercise).

—Do not make a scissors movement with the legs; during their alternating movement one of them remains in the vertical position.

—Do not fall heavily without controlling your return to the ground.

—During your return, do not let your head leave the carpet, which it touches throughout the exercise.

—Do not separate the legs; feet and knees should stay together while the posture is being taken up; they should only separate during the dynamic stage, and the legs must be lowered in the same way as they were raised.

—Do not push the chin towards the sternum, but apply the sternum to the chin.

—Do not get up suddenly when the posture is over (see 'Counter-posture' below).

FOR BEGINNERS

In the first stages people who find difficulty in carrying out Sarvān-gāsana because they are heavily built may first practise Ardha Sarvāngāsana (the half-shoulder-stand). In this the legs should be raised perpendicularly as before, then try to lift the trunk vertically, by supporting it with your hands under the buttocks, bending the knees to assume the position illustrated below. Then gradually raise the legs to an upright position to reach the normal asana. Never force the exercise, but practise it every day.

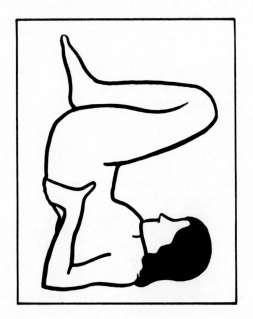

SUBSEQUENT POSTURE AND COUNTERPOSTURE

When Sarvāngāsana is integrated into a series of asanas, it precedes Halāsana (the Plough) which reinforces its effects.

When practised in isolation, it should be followed by its counter-posture 'Matsyāsana' (the Fish) which frees the neck and compresses the nape instead of stretching it. Ten respirations in Matsyāsana are enough to counterbalance Sarvāngāsana, even when the latter has lasted for several minutes.

FREQUENCY AND LENGTH OF PERFORMANCE

The Westerner who studies yogic literature may be put off by the differing opinions of its authors as to the frequency of practice, which varies from several times a day to only once, with the recommended time taken varying between a few seconds up to twenty minutes!

Who is right and what is the real truth? In one sense all of them are right! It is enough to realize that there are many ways in which Sarvāngāsana and yoga in general may be practised.

The 'full-time' Hindu yogi leads a very different life from the Western adept, and may practise several times a day, holding the posture for as long as twenty minutes. But the Westerner, who may have only half an hour in the day to spare for yoga, can only spend two or three minutes on this particular asana, and this is a good average time.

At the outset you may limit the time to a few seconds, and gradually increase it. Common sense is your best guide. It is a good thing to practise twice a day: the first time in the morning for the daily session, and then sometime during the day, or just before going to bed. It often helps one to fall asleep more rapidly and deeply: you should try it.

Do not allow 'time' to become an obsession! Your own organism should dictate the length: we are slaves to the clock during the entire day, let us at least escape it for our yoga session. It is better to count your respirations, so that you do not forget to breathe – something which can occur more easily than you may imagine!

CONTRA-INDICATIONS

At first sight these should correspond to those in the head-stand for which Sarvāngāsana may be substituted, but many people, although they cannot stand on their heads (there may be a delicate neck structure or vertebrae liable to displacement in the cervical region), can still practise Sarvāngāsana without risk.

There are few contra-indications in this asana, apart from severe ailments of the head and neck: otitis, dental abscess, angina, thyroid defects, sinusitis, sclerosis of the blood vessels of the brain, etc.

BENEFICIAL EFFECTS:
Generally speaking, many of the advantages of Sarvāngāsana are similar to those of Shīrṣāsana (see page 188). For instance:
    Improvement in the circulation of the blood (legs, stomach).
—Decongestion of the organs in the lower part of the stomach with relief from haemorrhoids.
—Relief in ptosis or prolapsus (of kidneys, stomach, intestines, uterus).
—Improvement in the flow of blood to the brain.
    These particular effects derive from its pronounced action on the thyroid gland, the thymus, and breathing.

The Spinal Column
Sarvāngāsana is entirely different from Shīrṣāsana in its effect upon the spinal column.

While the posture is being practised, it rids the spinal column of the curvatures normally present, which cause it to resemble a very elongated S (especially in the variant of this posture–see photograph on p. 107) while the cervical section of the column is stretched and flattened against the ground, serving to correct faults in the general deportment of the spine.

The Muscles
Sarvāngāsana strengthens the muscles of the abdomen, especially when it is practised with intermediary pauses when the legs are at 30° and 60°.

The Brain and Nervous System
Sarvāngāsana acts upon the cervical section of the spinal column, where the network of nerves, especially prolific in this region, is freed, toned up and generally revived. The substantial increase in the supply of blood to the brain under gentle pressure irrigates it, ridding it of the vascular spasms so often responsible for headaches.

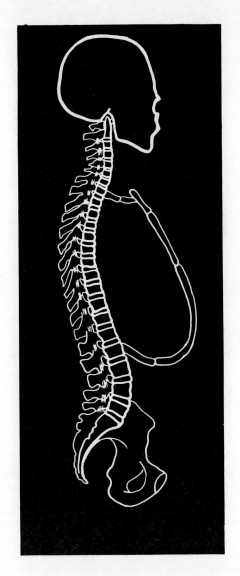

Upright deportment.
The spine is shaped like an elongated S.

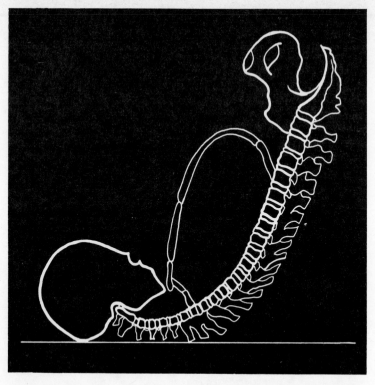

Sarvāngāsana smoothes out these curvatures, and by positioning the sternum against the chin, prevents movements of the thoracic cage, enforcing abdominal breathing.

The Endocrine Glands

The inverted posture and special position of the neck which accentuates the bend in the carotid artery, acts together with the compression induced in the region of the thyroid gland, to produce substantial irrigation. By this means Sarvāngāsana balances the slight functional changes in the thyroid, which are present in almost everyone. This slight hyper- or hypo-function, although not pathological, always has a definite effect on the metabolism. Since it acts upon the thyroid gland. Sarvāngāsana influences our behaviour, as well as all the functions of the body: hypo-thyroid subjects tend to be slow, heavy and indolent; hyperthyroids, on the other hand (and there are many of them!) breathe too rapidly and superficially, are subject to tachycardia, intestinal spasm and 'their manner of speaking is often an incomprehensible chatter' (Yesudian). Normalization of the thyroid induces calm, self-assurance, and as long as you do not overeat, it stabilizes the weight. The hypophysis or pituitary body, together with the hypothalamus, are thought to govern the hormonal production of the other endocrine glands, and these are also stimulated, which completes the effects of this posture on the head. Sarvāngāsana likewise affects the thymus, on which the growth of the body depends, and whose psychical and physical importance is vital in the development of both children and adolescents.

Breathing

The pressure of the sternum against the chin inhibits breathing from the top of the lungs and limits thoracic movements, so that the breathing automatically becomes diaphragmatic. It is therefore not surprising that Sarvāngāsana should produce beneficial effects in certain forms of asthma, and the posture is taught to adolescents suffering from this defect in respiration. A friend of mine, long an adept of yoga, told me that his son—an asthma sufferer—spent some time in a Swiss establishment where Sarvāngāsana and the head-stand were taught to young asthmatics. The asthmatic breathes through the top of the lungs, raising his shoulders; in Sarvāngāsana this form of breathing is impossible and he is therefore automatically forced to breathe from the abdomen. Moreover the viscera press on the diaphragm, aiding expiration and restoring mobility to this organ, which, in the asthmatic, is immobilized.

Another friend, who practises yoga despite long-standing asthma, suppresses its critical stages at their birth by means of Sarvāngāsana and yogic breathing: that is why the asana is such a valuable adjunct in medical therapy.

The Abdominal Organs

Sarvāngāsana helps to remedy ptosis or prolapsus, and drains the abdomen, ridding it of blood stases in the viscera, and eliminating at least temporarily, congestion in the lower abdomen: it aids the prostate gland as well!

Circulation of the Blood

The effects of Sarvāngāsana as a whole are similar to those of the head-stand. We should particularly notice the favourable reactions on the veins of the leg (preventing varicose veins) and on piles. Those who suffer from these afflictions, should practise the posture several times a day, (perhaps twice or three times) even when fully dressed, in addition to the medical treatment they are receiving. Sarvāngāsana is specially recommended to people whose work demands long hours of standing.

Aesthetic Effects

The posture brings a plentiful supply of blood to the face, especially to the forehead, where the skin at once becomes pink. It prevents, and even helps to dispel, wrinkles. Sarvāngāsana increases the blood supply to the scalp and nourishes the roots of the hair.

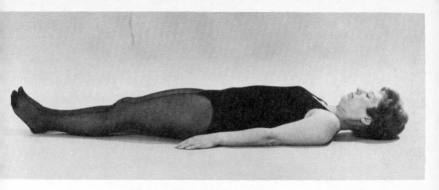

Starting position: identical to the Plough. Breathe calmly, bring the chin in towards the sternum, so as to prepare the nape of the neck to lie flat on the ground. The feet are together while the legs are not tensed. Before beginning to raise the feet, make sure the bottom of the back is touching the floor.

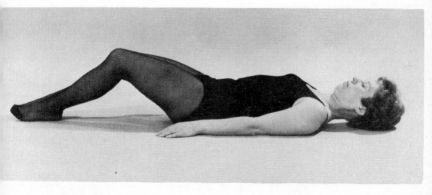

If you are unable to attain the posture, bend the knees a little.

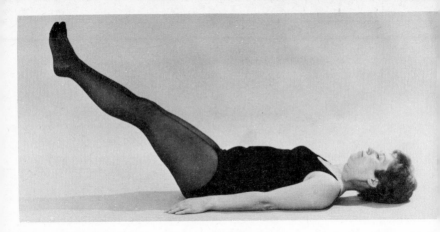

The legs are raised slowly. Meanwhile, it is essential to keep the whole length of the ba on the floor, especially in the lumbar region, so as to avoid any undue stress. Continue norm breathing. Do not tense the legs (the calves, and the underside of the thighs). Do not poi the feet. Relax the face, do not tense the arms; the stomach muscles are the ones which a going to carry out the movement. A pause may be made during the raising of the legs – t first at 30° and another at 60°.

Even during the pauses continue to breathe normally.

Bring the legs to the vertical position. Up to this point, the Plough and Sarvāngāsa are identical.

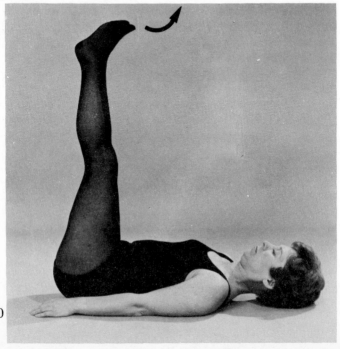

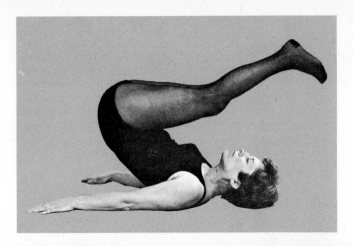

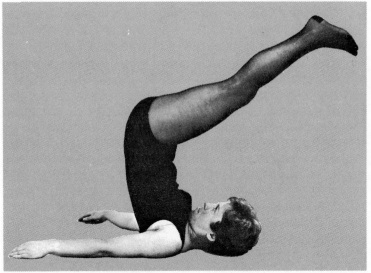

Above:
Begin to raise the buttocks from the floor. Inevitably at this point the leg-muscles will be tensed. Raise the feet up vertically above the head; continue to breathe calmly. Beginners may help themselves to lift the buttocks, by placing the hands under the hips.

Below:
Raise the feet slowly and bring the legs up as nearly as possible to the vertical. Do not tense the neck, but allow the nape to flatten onto the floor and the sternum to rise to touch the chin. Do not stop the breathing. Relax the calf and thigh muscles; therefore take care not to point the toes

101

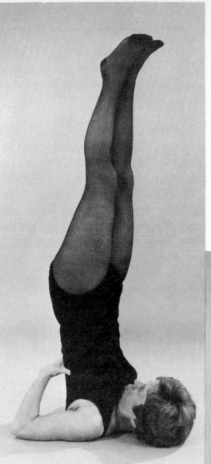

Correct final position, to be used as the starting position for the dynamic stage as well as at the static stage, when the position is maintained. The trunk is held as nearly vertical as possible, taking care not to tense the feet, and the legs are relaxed. The sternum is pressed against the chin, the nape of the neck is stretched and clings to the floor.

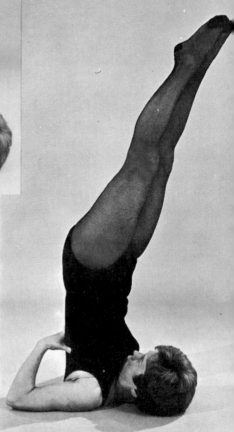

FAULT
The feet are pointed, which has produced tension in the legs.

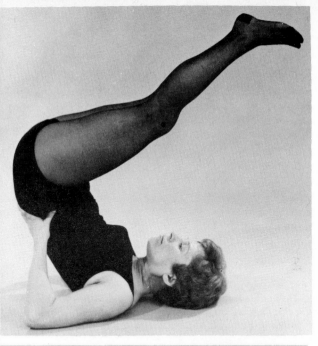

FAULT
The trunk should be more vertical. The sternum does not press on the chin, and there is therefore no direct action on the thyroid. This position may, however, serve for beginners.
To correct it:
Lower the hands and push with the forearms so as to erect the trunk. Do not tense the neck and its nape, which should be stretched and laid on the floor.

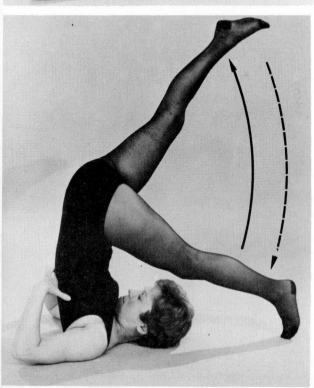

First stage of the dynamic phase
Keeping one leg still, allow the other to fall by its own weight to the floor. Breathe freely. Relax the thighs and calves. Now bring up the other leg to join the first which has been vertical. Work in this way alternating the right and left legs.

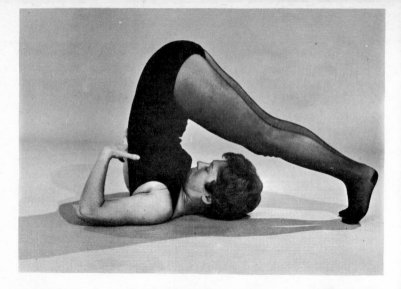

Now let the two feet down together. The force of their own weight will bring them to the floor. Do not tense the legs, but continue to breathe evenly. Do not immobilise the body when the toes have touched the ground, but return to the highest position, from which the static stage now begins (see photograph).

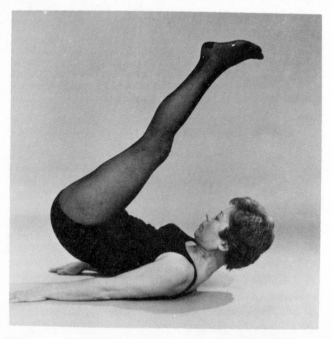

FAULT
Return to the floor in the opposite direction to the ascent. When so doing, take care to avoid letting the buttocks fall heavily and do not allow the nape to leave the ground.

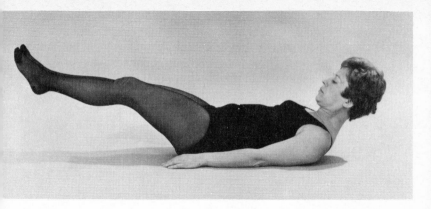

FAULT
The mistake made here is not uncommon: in returning the back too heavily to the ground, the legs have fallen with it, bringing the head up from the floor. The descent must be slow and controlled throughout.

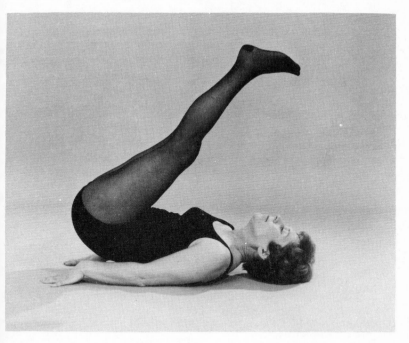

Beginners who are unable to bring the legs up vertically without bending the knees, may do so and (if necessary with the help of the hands supporting the buttocks), may begin with the position shown above.

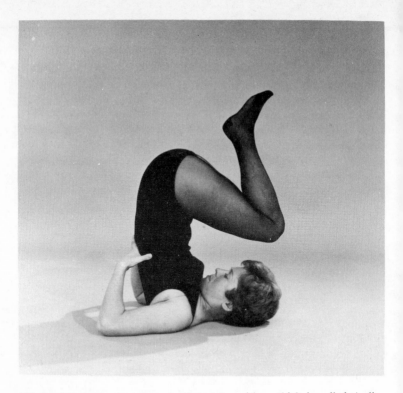

The beginner now passes on to the next position which is called Ardha-Sarvāngāsana (that is half-Sarvāngāsana). He can then bring the legs back and reach the final position without much trouble.

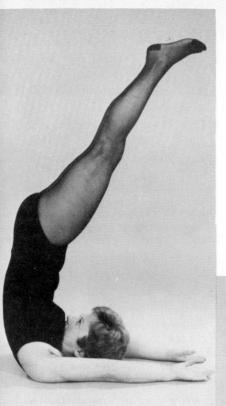

A Starting point as in Paschimottānāsana; that is with the arms stretched out behind the head.

VARIANTS OF THE FINAL POSITION

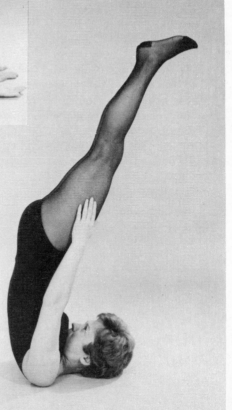

B Without any support, and by means of an abdominal contraction alone, bring up the legs and trunk to a vertical position, without jolting or sudden thrusting.

17. *Halāsana: The Plough*

Halāsana means the Plough posture. It is one of the only—if not the only—asana linked by name to a tool; in this case the primitive plough of ancient India.

The Yogis generally favour animal or insect names (Cobra, Locust, Peacock, etc.). This is one of the main postures in the group based on forward bending.

STARTING POSITION

(a) *For beginners:* begin by lying on the back, hands at the sides of the body, palms on the floor.

(b) *For advanced pupils:* as above, but the arms are stretched out behind the head, with the backs of the hands on the ground (see photograph, p. 114).

(c) *For the most advanced adepts:* as above, but the hands are joined under the back of the head (see photograph, p. 114).

In *each* case, before beginning the movement it is important, with the help of the hands, to stretch the neck and bring it as close as possible to the ground, bringing the chin in towards the chest, which assists the movement and compresses the thyroid more thoroughly in the final stage. The spinal column must be as flat as possible on the floor, especially in the lumbar region. If the curvature of the spine is so pronounced that you are unable to touch the floor, then bend the legs so that the loins touch the carpet, thus avoiding any displacement and helping you to master the posture.

TO CARRY OUT THE POSTURE

Halāsana is divided into two distinct parts: (a) a dynamic stage and (b) a static stage.

(A) THE DYNAMIC STAGE

This stage includes three procedures whereby the spinal column is

108

unwound in successive stages *throughout its length*. It precedes the period of immobilization which constitutes the asana itself and it is taken up in the following manner:

1. From either one of the three starting positions already described raise the legs to the vertical position, in a single, slow and continuous movement[1], without either hurrying or slowing it down.
2. By contracting the abdominal muscles, and keeping the legs straight, draw up the thighs to the chest, to release the lower part of the back. Towards the end of the movement, bend the legs a little so that the knees just brush the face.
3. Stretch out the legs and allow the feet to sink as far as possible to the ground so that in distancing themselves from the head the curvature of the back is accentuated. The upper part of the spine, particularly the nape of the neck, is thus bent.

RETURNING TO THE GROUND

Having pushed the feet out as far as possible from the head, without straining, continue without stopping – returning to the starting position in the same manner, but working in the opposite order. Do not allow the legs to fall back heavily, nor the head to come up from the ground.

As in every yogic movement, contract the minimum number of muscles; do not use more than is absolutely necessary. Pointing the feet can set up tension in the legs; instead the feet should hang as if weighted. *Repeat three times,* relaxing briefly between the movements.

Beginners may use their hands to help raise the buttocks, but must not succumb to the temptation of using a thrust to bring the feet behind the head. It is better to achieve this aim a month later than to use force or undue violence.

(B) THE STATIC STAGE

Normal Period of Development

The static stage constitutes the asana as such and consists, when

[1] Some yogis make a pause when the legs have reached an angle of 30° with the ground, followed by a second pause at 60°. Duration is for 2 to 3 respirations in each case. These pauses are optional and are reserved for advanced adepts.

the third unfolding movement has been completed, in keeping the body motionless in the final position attained at the end of the dynamic stage, and maintaining it thus for the prescribed length of time. Keep *strictly* motionless avoiding the slightest movement, relax, and allow the weight of the legs to stretch the spinal column.

Advanced Stage

The more advanced adept, having held the normal posture for five to ten breaths, should now bend the legs and bring the knees to the ears, sliding the hands behind the knees and the nape of the neck. Proceed, one hand at a time, while the other helps in preserving the balance. Set the elbows apart, and push them towards the ground so as to accentuate the bend of the spinal column. Should you wish, you may stretch the arms out behind the back and thrust out the palms, so that the body takes on the shape of an Ω (Omega).

RETURNING TO THE GROUND
In the reverse manner.

DURATION
When Halāsana is being done as part of a series of asanas, that is with a normal yoga session, the period of immobilisation lasts for from five to ten normal respirations, without holding the breath.

Beginners should limit themselves to five breaths and gradually increase the number as and when they progress sufficiently. When a yogi practises Halāsana (or indeed any other posture) in self-disciplined isolation, the exercise may last for fifteen or even thirty minutes! Certain authors (von Cyrass is one) mention this time without explaining that it is only for the most advanced. And this can lead to confusion. In disciplined conditions the difficulty is not to maintain the posture, since after a little practice it is comfortable, but rather to keep the absolute stillness required; after a few minutes, the mind begins to protest! Try to hold it for five minutes, and you will see! Remember the definition of an asana: any position which is assumed and maintained in immobility for a long time without undue effort, constitutes an asana.

BREATHING
Throughout the exercise, the breathing remains *normal* and must not be constrained or checked at any time, even while the legs are

being raised. Breathing should continue independently in its normal rhythm. When the knees are bent it is possible to breathe deeply so as to increase the abdominal massage.

CONCENTRATION
This, as we know, is the essential part of yoga. More, it is one of the basic differences between yoga and Western gymnastics which are carried out mechanically, without concentrated attention on the movements. Yoga, on the other hand, requires the attention to be persistently focused on the exercise; the mind is to the fore, all the body must do is to follow and obey.
During the dynamic stage concentrate upon carrying out the movement correctly and slowly, without jerking, and be sure to relax all the muscles concerned.
During the static stage focus the concentration either on the breathing (this for beginners who will find they tend to 'forget' to breathe) or on the absolute immobility required, or again upon the spinal column and the neck, where the thyroid lies (this for advanced adepts).

FAULTS
—Bending the knees during the actual asana, except at the moment prescribed.
—Straining; you must work gently without jerking. Proceed gradually, taking care not to tire yourself. Take your time and relax the muscles.
—If you strain a muscle you may have to wait for a few weeks before you can take up the exercise again.
—Contracting the shoulders, the jaws or the neck.
—Breathing insufficiently may induce a feeling of suffocation.

ADVICE TO BEGINNERS
The spinal column is loosened by the weight of the legs. Wait until the toes, as an outcome of this traction, lower themselves gradually and of their own accord until they touch the floor. Remain calm and relaxed. At the beginning you may feel uncomfortable in this position (the breathing may be restricted if the stomach is of any size) but this soon improves.

111

The real essential is daily correct practice carried out with patience and without haste. You should keep the mind disengaged and treat outside factors as if viewing them from afar.

CONTRA-INDICATIONS

It is helpful to remember that yoga begins where medicine ends. In other words, anyone suffering from an acute condition should wait for it to be cured before beginning to practise yoga. If you are in doubt, consult your doctor. During menstruation, women should avoid any attempt to force the exercise, especially in the stage where the abdominal region is compressed. They should show reasonable care but should not shrink from practising the exercise.

Those suffering from a serious or a strangulated hernia, should not attempt it.

BENEFICIAL EFFECTS

This asana acts as a powerful tonic, for it works upon the entire spinal column, which contains and protects the spinal cord, and which is furthermore bordered by the dense network of ganglia and their fibres, the lateral chain influencing the sympathetic nervous system, which affects the automatic functions of the body. It is therefore not difficult to see why this asana is so rejuvenating and reviving.

The stretching of the back muscles expels the blood, which is then replaced by a fresh influx. The important neighbouring nerve centres benefit from this. The flexibility of the spinal column—which is so essential to health—is restored and protected by this posture. The abdominal muscles are reinforced, because they initiate the movement during the dynamic·stage, and there are innumerable good effects, deriving from healthy abdominal muscles and the maintenance of the viscera in the correct position.

Under compression the thyroid gland benefits from an increased flow of fresh blood, which helps to regularise its functions. By controlling the metabolism, this gland has a considerable influence on the youthfulness of the body, and by secreting hormones acts upon various other glands, as well as upon the intestines, blood pressure, the mobility of migratory cells (the white corpuscles which fight infection), and stimulates the nervous system. Hyperthyroid conditions lead to irritability and underweight. This exercise, therefore, serves to calm the nerves by contributing to the normal function of the thyroid. Conversely, when that gland fails to produce sufficient hormones, the metabolism is slowed down, the skin becomes wrinkled and dry, the blood pressure drops too low, and there is an insufficiency of sexual activity, together with both physical and mental laziness. Halāsana is an excellent therapy in such cases, but if there are *pathological* changes in the thyroid gland, it is necessary to consult a doctor. In the majority of cases the indications given above are only relevant to small deviations from the normal condition.

The slow unwinding of the spinal column involves each of the vertebrae and constitutes an ideal orthopaedic exercise. This posture is very reviving. When you are tired in the evening, all you have to do is to devote a minute or two to it, and you will quickly be yourself again. Because the body is in the inverted position, arterial blood flows towards the head and irrigates the brain better. The face receives an extra supply, especially over the forehead and the scalp – all excellent in helping to prevent lines and wrinkles.

Apart from its action on the thyroid gland, this posture has a good effect on the spleen and the sexual glands, especially in its final stage when the legs are bent with the thighs pressing on the stomach, thus reducing the space available for the abdominal organs, and compressing them; the blood is pressed along and stoppages are eliminated. The organ especially affected is the liver, which is cleansed, decongested and stimulated. Moreover the slightest state of congestion or blood stasis in the liver has an immediate effect on the function of the whole digestive tract. The pancreas is likewise massaged, purified and toned up. There are cases in which diabetics have been able to reduce their daily intake of insulin, or have even managed to rid themselves completely of the disease, which is easily explained if we realize that the pancreas contains the Islets of Langerhans, which produce insulin.

This asana fights constipation, which is the hidden cause of innumerable ills, it effectively reduces cellulitis and overweight by improving the function of the alimentary canal, normalising the metabolism, and massaging any adipose tissue strongly in the final stage.

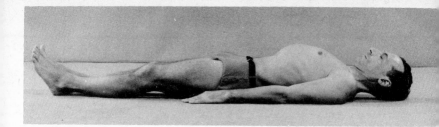

Starting position for beginners. Notice the position of the head (the chin is tucked inwards).

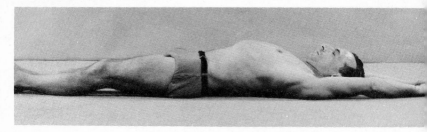

Starting position for pupils with some degree of proficiency. The back, nape of the neck and the arm all lie as straight as possible in line one with another!

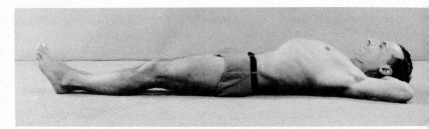

Starting position for advanced adepts.

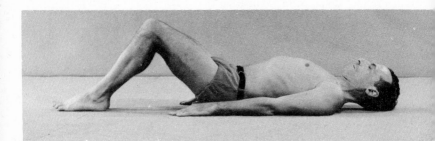

If the beginner is unable to make the back touch the floor when his legs are stretched out, he may begin the posture with his knees bent. This applies also to the return.

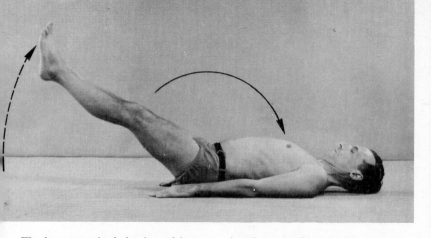

The legs are raised slowly and kept as relaxed as possible; the feet *must not be pointed*. The back is laid firmly along the ground in order to avoid any misalignment in the loins (this is important). Raise the legs slowly in one continuous movement, until they reach the vertical position. The return takes place in the same manner.

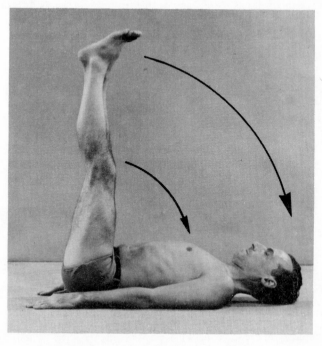

Bring the legs up to the vertical position.

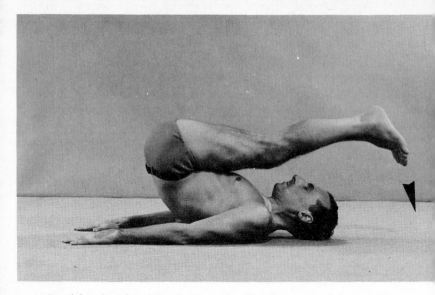

By tightening the abdominal muscles (for they control the movement), bring the thighs up as closely as possible to the chest, so as to bend the *base* of the spinal column.

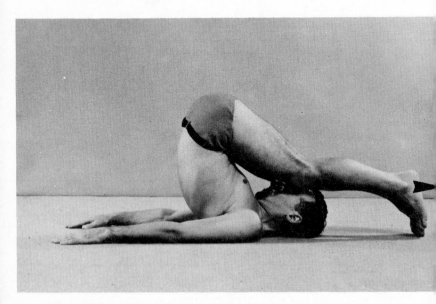

The unfolding of the spine takes place by bringing the knees up to the face. At this point the legs are *slightly* bent.

116

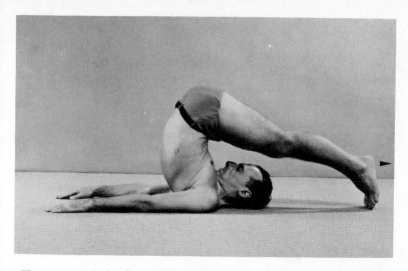

The toes touch the floor. With each exhalation they should be pushed slowly back as far as possible. This completes the unwinding of the spine, by acting upon the dorsal region and the cervicals of the vertebral column.

Static stage I: a minimum of five breaths.
The legs are relaxed. If they do not reach the floor at first, wait until they bear down with their own weight. No jerky movements should be allowed.

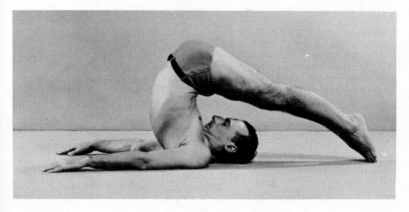

FAULT
The feet are pointing backwards, which means that the thighs, calves, and even the base of the back are all forced to contract.

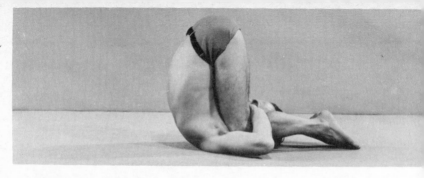

Static stage II: Of average difficulty.
The knees are bent, the hands are placed at the backs of the knees, and serve as support at the nape of the neck.
Breathe deeply (the massage of the viscera is very intense). Do not miss out the static stage. Bring the chin well into the chest and press the nape against the ground.

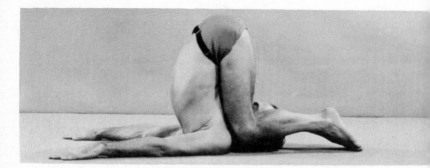

Static stage III: Of average difficulty.
This is optional after stage II. Advanced pupils carry out the three stages accompanied by for example, five respirations at each position.

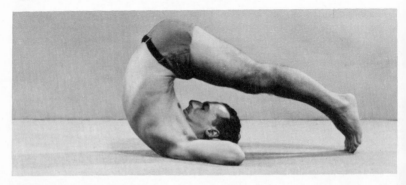

This static stage is only for advanced adepts who have used the most elaborate of the starting positions. There is great tension in the nape of the neck. Throughout the movement both reaching the posture and on return, the elbows must remain in contact with the floor.

18. *Matsyāsana: The Fish*[1]

There is a curious origin to the strange and exotic name given to an asana which does not in any way appear fishlike! The Sanskrit texts maintain – with some justification – that it allows one to float in water like a fish. In the classic 'float' the face emerges barely enough to allow one to breathe, while in the Fish posture it is far enough out of the water to remain untouched by any but the roughest wave. In effect, Matsyāsana increases the capacity to float by moving the centre of gravity towards the middle of the body, allowing improved ventilation of the lungs.

COUNTER-POSTURE TO SARVĀNGĀSANA AND HĀLASANA
However it is not for its seaworthy qualities that we are about to study this posture! In fact, it forms the counter-posture to Sarvān-gāsana and Halāsana which stretch the cervical region, and in which the chin, closely pressed to the sternum, compresses the thyroid, simultaneously preventing any expansion of the thorax. During these two postures, therefore, any deeper thoracic or clavicular breathing is out of the question. It is essential to counter-balance their action; which is why Matsyāsana is placed directly after them.

Matsyāsana arches the nape, frees and stretches the neck, removes the compression which the thyroid gland has undergone (to its distinct advantage), assists thoracic and clavicular breathing, and stretches the abdomen.

METHOD
Matsyāsana in its classic form is taken up in the Lotus position and carried out in this fashion so as to allow the body to float. Since the Lotus is inaccessible to many Westerners – and not only to beginners – there is, fortunately, a variant within the scope of everyone, the effects of which are in practice identical to those of the classical asana. This is the posture we are about to describe:

[1] Matsya means 'fish' in Sanskrit

First of all, sit on the ground with your legs stretched out in front.

First Phase
Leaning the trunk slightly back and to the right, place the right and then the left elbow on the floor and lean on them.

Second Phase
Push the chest forwards and up leaning the head backwards as far as possible, so that you see 'the world upside down'. Hollow the back as much as possible by arching yourself from the elbows.

NOTE: In rare cases (generally in those subject to sea and air sickness) this head position induces nausea and giddiness. These handicaps are related to a defect in the middle ear, which is irreversible – where this is so, there is nothing to be gained by further trial: this asana should be given up, and replaced within the session by one or two minutes' relaxation, accompanied by deep breathing.

FINAL POSITION
Lower the head to the floor, moving the elbows forward. Hollow the back as completely as possible so that it forms an arch supported at one end by the top of the head and at the other by the buttocks, with the elbows acting as support in between.

When he first practises this posture the student should stop at this point: later when he finds the posture easy, he may place his hands on his thighs, which means he can forego the elbows' support.

DURATION
Hold the posture for ten deep breaths.

RETURNING TO THE GROUND
The return is carried out by relaxing the back so as to lie flat on the floor, and not by reversing the direction used in taking up the posture; rest for a few seconds in this position.

BREATHING
Respiration must be as high as possible in the body, near the collar-

bones. In Matsyāsana the trachea (windpipe) is opened widely, which provides a good opportunity to ventilate the apex of the lungs thoroughly. Separate the ribs well while you are raising the shoulder-blades. Abdominal breathing is reduced, which is both desirable and required.

When breathing out, contract the muscles which serve to lower the ribs and bring them together, thus emptying the lungs completely. Finally tighten the abdominal muscles, so as to expel the remaining air from the lungs.

REPETITION
When placed within a series of asanas, a single performance is enough, but should you be able to spare some minutes, it is advisable to repeat it a second time. It is better, however, to run through it twice in succession than to attempt to try and lengthen the time in which you hold it, because the back will arch with greater ease at the second attempt.

CONCENTRATION
Alternately upon the tensed muscular structure of the back, and then on the deep respiration through the top of the lungs.

FAULT
The buttocks should not be raised from the floor – a frequent mistake.

CLASSIC POSTURE
Except for the starting position, the preceding instructions apply also to those who will eventually be able to take up the Lotus posture. One more difference lies in the final position, when the feet are held in the hands so as to exert traction, thus accentuating the curve in the loins and increasing the effectiveness of the posture.

BENEFICIAL EFFECTS
As a counter-posture Matsyāsana fully ensures the complete effectiveness of Sarvāngāsana and Halāsana by balancing its action. Furthermore Matsyāsana produces specially good effects upon the thorax (chest), spinal column and abdominal region.

Thorax and Lungs

Matsyāsana has a specially good effect on the thorax.

In childhood we are compelled to sit on school benches or at a desk, and these enforced hours of immobilization lead in many cases to restriction of the thorax, so that the ribs, instead of remaining normally placed, are slanted in relation to the spine, and in this way the space occupied by the lungs–that is their vital capacity–is reduced, and normal breathing becomes impossible; a fact which detracts from our vitality and health. If you carry out Uḍḍiyāna in front of the glass, you will see your ribs standing out. In some people their ribs are wrongly set in the form of a Gothic arch; if the ribs form a dome, then the chest is normal. In 'Gothic' cases Matsyāsana is a benediction and sufferers are well advised to practise it assiduously, if necessary several times a day, even outside their normal daily sessions of yoga. Measure the circumference of your chest at the last point of the breast bone (the xiphoid cartilage). Six weeks later check this measurement, and you will be convinced and encouraged by the improvement. The lungs being joined with the thorax, your vital capacity will likewise have increased to the same extent. During the asanas the upper lobes, and more especially the region under the collar-bones will receive more air.

The Spinal Column

A restricted thorax is often accompanied by a round, stiffened back, especially near the shoulder blades: Matsyāsana has a direct effect on this disfavoured region.

At the start some people will have great difficulty, however ultimately worthwhile the effort, in achieving the Fish posture. They must not be depressed, because patient determination *will* succeed and the game is worth the candle.

Muscles

Matsyāsana is particularly good for strengthening the muscles of the spine. The back is flushed by the increased supply of blood, and a pleasant warmth is felt. The asana also acts upon the abdominal wall, which it stretches without in any way distending it.

The Nervous System

The plentiful supply of blood to the back muscles of which we have spoken, spreads through to the spinal cord, which increases the vital elasticity by the natural and gentle stimulation of each of the essential workings of the body. It likewise has good effects upon the sympathetic nervous system. The region of the solar plexus is often beset by perpetual spasm, caused through the constant anxiety which arises from the frenzied lives we lead; through the stretching of the abdomen and the deepened breathing, the region becomes decongested.

Abdominal Viscera

This stretching of the abdomen, together with the internal massage brought about by deep breathing, likewise tones up the viscera in the abdominal cavity: the liver and spleen are among the beneficiaries. It is an excellent posture for women, because it stimulates the organs in the pelvis, especially the genital ones and in particular the ovaries.

Matsyāsana alleviates painful or bleeding haemorrhoids, without of course dispensing with the need for appropriate medical treatment which the asana assists considerably.

The Endocrine Glands

We have just referred to the special significance of the asana in assisting the genital glands, thus improving hormone secretion. The adrenals are toned up and the production of adrenalin and cortisone is normalized; there is no risk of these overstepping their normal level of production. The posture, in stimulating the pancreas, helps in cases of false diabetes of nervous origin.

Its Aesthetic Effects

Matsyāsana remodels the chest and straightens the back, ensuring a proper posture, which in turn has its effects on the psychological make-up.

The Special Effects of the Classic Posture

The advantages already mentioned are equally applicable to the classic asana. In addition, the Lotus posture slows down the circulation by compressing the femoral artery in the thighs, to some extent diverting its flow of blood from the legs into the base of the stomach. Men benefit most from this effect on the gonads. Matsyāsana is therefore a posture with particularly reviving qualities.

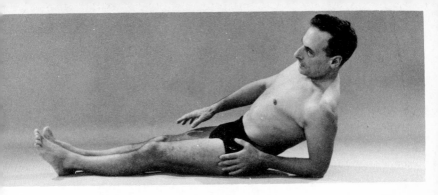

From a sitting position with legs stretched in front, place first one and then the other elbow on the floor for support.

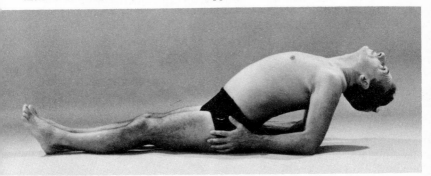

When both elbows have touched the ground, lean the head backwards hollowing the small of the back as much as possible. Then . . .

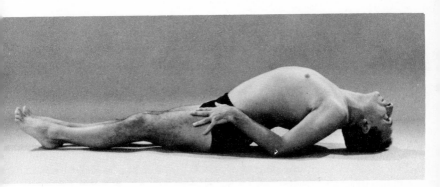

. . . rest the head on the floor. The elbows may remain there at first so as to furnish an intermediary support to the arch formed by the back. This arch is supported at one end by the top of the head, at the other by the buttocks.

Because the trachea is opened up, it is necessary to breathe deeply, so as fully to ventilate the upper lobes of the lungs.

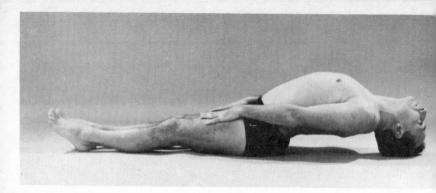

Now place the hands on the thighs: this makes the posture harder but because the central support of the elbows has been removed, the exercise is made more effective.

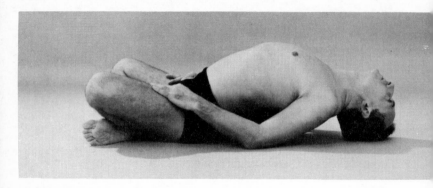

The posture shown above may be practised for Sukhāsana, the easy posture, otherwise known as the tailor posture.

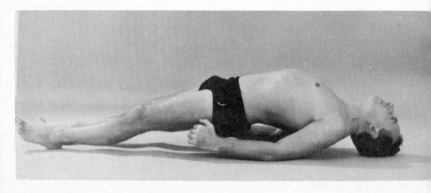

FAULT Avoid lifting the buttocks from the floor.

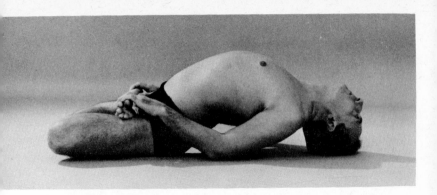

The classic position begins in the Lotus posture which, unfortunately many Westerners are unable to attain. The photograph was taken when the lungs were inflated to their maximum which would allow the body to float easily on water, without any additional movement.

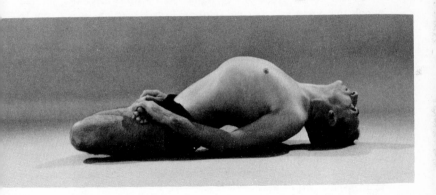

This photograph differs from the previous one in a single detail of respiration. After exhaling, empty the lungs completely, by pulling in the abdominal muscles as shown here.

19. *Pashchimottānāsana: The Forward Bend*

No, your eyes are not deceiving you!

'*Pashchi*mottānāsana' is translated in an extraordinarily different number of ways. It may seem trifling to linger over its exact meaning, since it is the posture and not the name that counts; the temptation is to leave such questions to learned Sanskritists, and to stick to the practical side, but this asana is a special case: it is essential to understand its exact meaning.

As you know, yogis like to name their asanas after the animals which the postures resemble (Cobra, Locust, etc.) as it is easier to memorize and identify them. So if Pashchimottānāsana is the exception, it is clearly not because the yogis lack the imagination to think up a suitable symbol.

Let us begin with the *anatomical* meaning:

'Pashchima' in Sanskrit means posterior, and 'tan' means extension or stretch—so that the literal translation is 'stretching (or lengthening) of the back'. One author considers there is not much wrong with the term 'extension of the posterior'! Others know it as 'the seated grip' to distinguish it from the 'standard grip' (Pāda-hastāsana), and since the term is conveniently short we are tempted to adopt it.

Pashchimottānāsana however, conceals a meaning which must be examined more closely. 'Pashchima' = the west; Paschimottānāsana therefore, should mean 'climbing westwards' which seems, and is, deliberately pointless and inexplicable to the uninitiated. Alain Daniélou has given us the key in his book *Yoga, the Way to Reintegration*, p. 50.

'When in this posture the subtle breath of life rises through the subtle central channel in the spine (Sushumnā) to reach the back of the head, it is said that it 'is ascending by the back way' (the West, Pashchima, Mārga), from whence it receives its name. But, when it rises through the subtle channel between the eyebrows to the uppermost region of the head, or 'the thousand-petalled lotus', it is said to follow the 'forward way' (the East, Pūrva, Mārga).

Whereas in the Posture of Self-Realization (Siddha-āsana) both channels of the subtle body, the East and West, are of equal import, in the present context the rear one becomes more important. Furthermore, when the breath of life passes through only one of the two subtle channels, more rapid results are obtained, which explains how especially valuable this posture is.'

METHOD

Starting Position
Lie on the back, arms stretched out as far as possible behind the head. Some writers advise starting from a sitting position; but this is inadvisable, because it lessens the effects considerably by cutting short the dynamic stage. Even the beginner should not fall back on this easy alternative, since it can only benefit the more intractable cases temporarily.

TAKING UP THE ASANA
The posture, like those of the Plough and the Cobra, contains a dynamic and a static stage.

DYNAMIC STAGE
This consists of three successive unwinding movements of the spinal column, carried out in succession to form a single, slow and continuous one.

First Phase
Lie on the back, arms stretched out behind the head. Breathe freely. Relax briefly, then slowly raise the arms to the vertical. The head should remain motionless on the floor. The thumbs are linked to ensure a bending movement in the axis of the body. The arm muscles are fully relaxed, so that they would not rise if the strength being used were curtailed in the slightest degree.

Second Phase
When the arms have reached the vertical, the arc of the circle

described by the hands moves towards the thighs; as the head and shoulders rise, the eyes are focused on the fingers, but the back remains on the floor—*very important.*

At this point look towards the knees.

Third Phase

As soon as the fingers have touched the thighs, push the hands towards the feet, lightly touching the shins on the way. The trunk is being raised to a sitting position from whence it begins to lean forward. It is essential to uncurl the whole length of the spine. You will see from the photographs how the movement is achieved in detail.

While the hands gradually· move towards the feet, the forehead is brought down to touch the knees, if possible, after which it presses forward, moving as close as possible to the feet. The body is now folded in two like a penknife. The chest rests against the legs. (See 'Advice to Beginners', p. 131.)

Return

Slowly return to the starting position, making sure that you uncurl the back in the opposite direction until you reach the ground. Do not remove the hands from the thighs until almost the whole of the back is on the carpet. Replace the arms behind the head.

These details are of great importance. If they are disregarded the exercise loses much·of its effect.

Repeat the above movement three times. This is the dynamic stage.

THE STATIC STAGE

This stage is at the end of the third unwinding movement, and contains two motionless periods:

First Immobilization:

In the 'crochet-hook' position (see photograph, p. 140) which is achieved as follows: Place the thumbs on the knee-caps, the other fingers under the knees, elbows into sides of the thighs (important). Bring the forehead as close as possible to the knees, while pushing the arms back (see arrows in the photograph) to bring the nose in towards the navel; tighten the abdomen so as to increase the curvature and stretching in the top of the back. Then breathe deeply five times.

Second Immobilization:
Let go of the knees; push the hands along the tibiae and catch hold of the toes; then pull steadily and slowly to bring the chest towards the knees. Try to stretch the spine as much as you can.

This is the final development; breathe deeply from five to ten times. The back should remain as motionless and relaxed as possible, throughout. The movement is made with the help of the abdominal muscles.

ADVANCED VARIANT
Advanced adepts place the feet apart, pointing the toes inwards and touching the ground with the forehead or chin. Hold the position still while breathing deeply (see photograph).

ADVICE TO BEGINNERS
At first it is sometimes uncomfortable to move on from the recumbent to the seated position; if so, you may cheat a little by bending the knees, and hooking your hands under them, or alternatively you may slide the feet beneath a piece of furniture. The spinal column will soon become more flexible and you will find you can raise yourself, at first with a little extra push, later without.

If the asana is to be performed perfectly, the legs must be kept straight and flat on the ground. This may at first prove impossible, so the *knees may be bent slightly,* which produces little effect on the curvature of the spine.

FAULTS
The most frequent errors are as follows:
—Raising the back before the hands touch the thighs. This means the spinal column does not uncurl properly.
—When the ankles are grasped to bring the forehead down to the feet, it is a mistake to make jerky, repetitive movements, as in physical training, since the back cannot remain passive and relaxed meanwhile: it is preferable not to try to reach any lower but to keep the movement smooth instead.

—Bending the knees.
—On the return, allowing the body to fall back without uncurling the spine.

DURATION
The immobilization period will vary a great deal according to whether it is being practised by a beginner or an advanced adept expert, and also whether within a series of asanas or in isolation.

(a) *Within a complete series:*
Final stage: five to ten complete and deep breaths is a good average.
(b) *As a single posture:*
Yogis advise holding the posture as long as possible (Dhirendra Bramachari in Delhi) without giving more precise instructions. Three to fifteen minutes is long enough for most people, as von Cyrass suggests. In this case the increased effects produce spectacular rejuvenating results in the body within a few months, although feats of this kind should not be rashly attempted in the absence of personal guidance from a qualified instructor.

The warning is somewhat superfluous, because the Westerner can seldom spare half-an-hour a day for his yoga!

BREATHING
In this as in every other exercise, breathing continues normally and freely at every stage, and must not be stopped at any time, especially when the trunk is rising from a lying to a seated position. When you are moving the forehead along to touch the feet, you will realize how much easier it is to exhale than to breathe in. During the final motionless period, make the most of every expiration and so make it easier to relax the back completely and if possible to stretch the spine, be it only a millimetre more.

CONCENTRATION
During the dynamic stage, you may concentrate either on the slow progressive movement or on relaxing the muscles of the back and on the breathing.

Although this posture stretches the back, the mind must concentrate on the solar plexus, *not* on the spinal column. During the static stage, however, you may concentrate on the base of the back.

General

The effects produced by the dynamic stage, differ from those of the static one which succeeds it.

The dynamic stage stimulates the whole nervous network along the spine: this is due to the slow unwinding procedure, which, besides conferring perfect mobility on the spine, tones up the whole organism, and reacts on the sympathetic ganglia located in paired chains along the spinal column from the skull to the coccyx. The abdominal muscles, which are employed to raise the trunk, are strengthened.

During the static stages, the effects derive from the compression of the abdomen by the thighs, which induces the abdominal muscles to tone up the viscera. Stimulation of the sympathetic and para-sympathetic systems of the pelvis is effected by stretching the base of the back, and this in turn reacts on the organic activity of the abdominal region. This asana removes excess fat from the stomach and the hips.

Spinal Column

Pashchimottānāsana and Halāsana complement each other and their action is closely associated: the static stage in Halāsana has a particular effect on the upper part of the spinal column, whereas Pashchimottānāsana tones up the lumbar region of the spine. During both asanas, the vertebrae separate gently from each other, and free the network of the nerves which emerge from the spinal cord.

The extensive stretching of the muscles in the grooves of the vertebrae forces blood from the muscles, which returns, increased in volume, and serves to irrigate the spinal cord.

The Muscles and Nervous System

The muscles in the region of the spinal column and the abdomen are strengthened. The stretching of muscles and ligaments, as well as the nerves in the back of the legs, alleviates certain cases of sciatica by freeing the nerve from its displaced position. In the final period of immobility, the solar plexus and the nervous system of the spine are gently stimulated and freed from congestion. All anxiety states are alleviated thereby and this is no surprise to a yoga expert who clearly understands the powerful effect asanas have upon the psyche, although the layman may remain unconvinced.

The Abdominal Viscera

The stimulating action of this asana affects every organ in the abdomen.

There is a marked effect upon the prostate gland, among others. Those whose sexual activity has begun to decline experience a renewal of vigour, but without unhealthy over-stimulation. Many adepts have referred to the re-awakening of their sexuality – and this at an advanced age – after prolonged inactivity. Psychologically, of course, this sign of renewed youth has a very favourable effect on the general balance and self-confidence; physically, reactivation of the gonads, whose hormone secretions are of such importance (Voronoff and many others have convinced us of this) has enormous repercussions on the health, and is responsible for some astonishing rejuvenating effects without recourse to gland extracts or grafts; the hormones are produced by the individual himself and these secretions are irreplaceable; this applies to men as well as to women, whose uterus and ovaries are benefited.

The pancreas, too, is stimulated and toned up by this asana; the liver, kidneys and bladder are all equally invigorated, and the peristaltic movements of the intestines increase, especially of the large intestine or colon; many intractable cases of constipation have been brought to an end, often only in a matter of days.

There are some people, however, who may increase their tendency to constipation if they hold the asana for more than five minutes. A little wisdom must be employed in any attempts to practise the longer immobilisation stages without an experienced guide.

The Lymphatic Circulation

Generally speaking, we are only interested in the circulation of blood. Yet it is very unwise to underestimate the importance of the lymph which helps to fight infection and which is greatly affected by yoga. When this circulation is slowed down, we are far more vulnerable to bacteria which can, in some cases, enter the lymph and find their way deep into the organism; this cannot occur when the lymphatic circulation is normal.

Effects on the Health

The salutary effects of this asana have been described in the preceding paragraphs. We shall list them once again:

This asana is specific in cases of: constipation, haemorrhoids, diabetes, dyspepsia, indigestion and poor appetite; it gets rid of numerous functional disorders of the liver, gall-bladder, kidneys, intestines, spleen and seminal secretions. It helps to alleviate enlargement of the liver and kidneys, and assists the stomach in proper evacuation; it also prevents certain forms of ulcer. It clears away lordosis.

Aesthetic Effects

The improvement of the spinal column corrects the posture, and the increased flexibility of the spine enhances grace in every movement. This asana, by ridding the body of adipose tissue over the stomach and thighs, improves the appearance. The figure fines down through the renewed strength in the abdominal muscles; the waist is reduced.

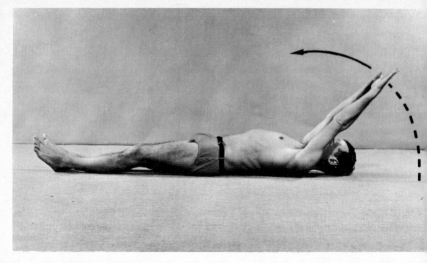

At the start of the exercise, only the arms are moved with a minimum of muscle power. Concentrate upon this arm movement. Breathe normally.

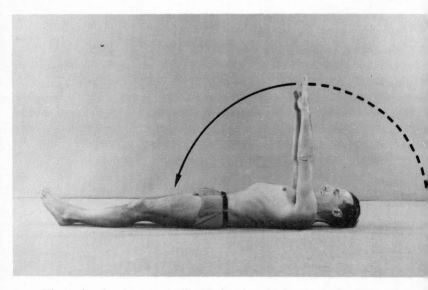

First raise the arms vertically. Notice that the head remains in constant contact with the ground. One detail to notice is that the thumbs are hooked together, so as to ensure symmetrical movement in relation to the body.

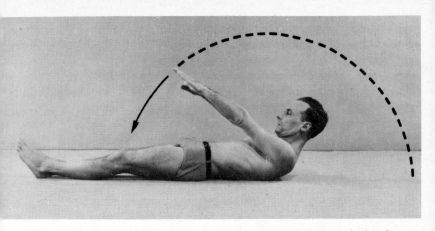

The hands continue to circle in an arc towards the thighs. Only the head and elbows leave the floor. The gaze is upon the tips of the fingers.

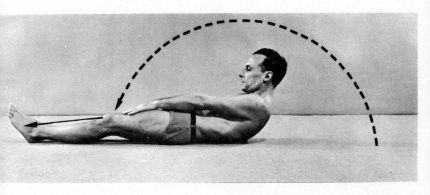

The hands touch the thighs. Most of the back remains touching the ground. The eyes are focused on the knees. The back gradually curves, and you will notice, if you watch how it uncurls throughout the dynamic stage, the moment at which each and every part of the spinal column is carefully stretched vertebra by vertebra.

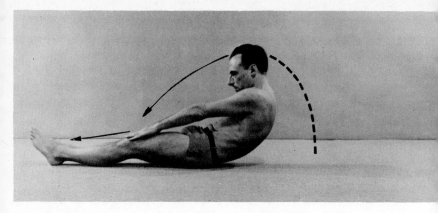

When the hands have come to touch the thighs, and *not before*, they are pushed towards the tibiae, and the back remaining as rounded as possible is raised from the floor.

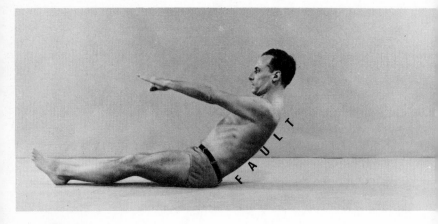

FAULT
The back rises before the hands have come to rest on the thighs, and therefore moves in one piece, rather than vertebra by vertebra. *This is a common fault.*

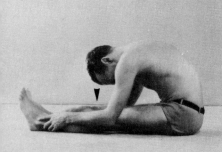

The head is brought down to the knees while the hands, in a single and slow movement, move towards the feet.

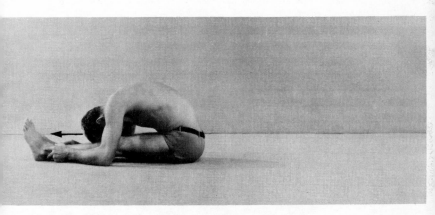

At this point, lower the forehead, if possible to touch the knees.

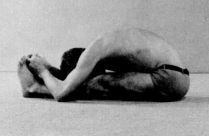

Now by taking hold of the big toes with the middle fingers, the thumbs hooked together, flatten the legs as much as possible so as to stretch the base of the spine to the utmost extent. The posture will then justify its significant name: 'the back-stretching posture'.

Return in the opposite direction, repeat three times and you have completed the dynamic stage of the asana.

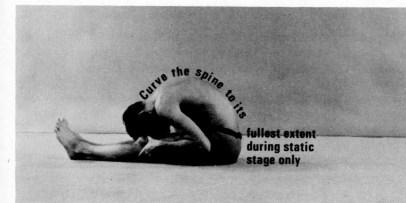

Curve the spine to its fullest extent during static stage only

At the third unwinding, you may, if you like, increase the curvature of the back, and hold it for a moment in the 'hook' position. The thumbs are on the kneecaps and the elbows press the body. The arms are pushed so as to bring the head back as near as possible to the knees and stomach; the latter is stiffened in order to curve the spine to the maximum degree.

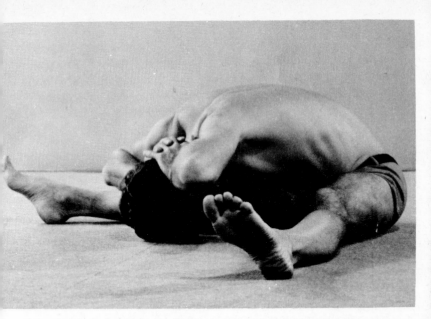

When they have completed the static stage, the more advanced adepts will increase the movement by placing the feet apart, and gradually but smoothly relaxing the muscles in the back and thighs, the head moving towards the floor, until the forehead touches the ground. At this juncture, breathe five to ten times. Notice how, in the angle formed by the legs, the feet are turned inwards rather than outwards.

20. *Bhujaṅgāsana: The Cobra*

This asana is known as the Cobra, because in it the adept raises the head and trunk together in a similar way to this reptile, which spreads its hood when it is roused (Bhujanga = Cobra in Sanskrit).

METHOD

Starting Point

In Halāsana there are various starting points from which to choose, whereas in the Cobra there is only one: it is not difficult to assume it correctly, but to do so is essential to the correct progression of the asana as a whole.

Lie flat on the abdomen, legs stretched out with feet together, the soles turned up. The arms are bent and the hands rest flat on the floor, the tips of the fingers in line with the top of the rounded shoulder (this is very important). The elbows are to the sides of the body. Lay the forehead on the floor before beginning the movements.

TAKING UP THE ASANA—THE DYNAMIC STAGE

Bhujaṅgāsana is simple; in it the head and trunk are raised as high as possible so that the spinal column is bent back. The performance of this asana entails an assortment of details which demonstrate how cultivated and perfect yoga techniques can be. Every detail has been proved to be essential and, one has only to omit a single one deliberately to realize how much the posture's effects are diminished. Before moving on to the method, it must be explained that in its dynamic stage Bhujaṅgāsana acts mainly upon the *upper* part of the spinal column, in the static stage, it acts upon the column as a whole.

First Stage

The adept lies flat on his stomach, forehead pressed to the ground.

After a second or two of relaxation, he slowly pushes the nose forward, skimming the ground: the chin follows, lightly brushing the carpet and pushing forward as far as possible. Then the neck is stretched, while the nape is compressed. Out of ignorance this first stage is sometimes skipped, which is unwise, because the cervical region of the spinal column is a strategic central stem from which numerous vital nerves branch out.

Second Stage
When the chin has been brought as far forward as possible, raise the head slowly in one smooth movement by contracting the muscles at the nape of the neck. Then the dorsal muscles are brought into action, so that *no help is given by the arms,* which remain relaxed. The weight of the arms rests on the palms of the hands which are, in turn, laid on the ground. The eyes look up to the ceiling as far as possible. When the dorsal muscles are thoroughly contracted, the legs, but not the calves, are tensed and the whole weight of the body rests on the stomach where the pressure increases. The back flushes demonstrating how great is the influx of blood into both the inner and the superficial dorsal regions.

Return
The return to the ground is carried out with the same care as the ascent. The mechanism to be used is the same but it works in the opposite sense. That is to say, first the arms gradually and slowly release their pressure, while the back and leg muscles remain relaxed. Where, at the start of the movement the arms were brought into action, now the back muscles take over the work, controlling the descent until the chin returns to the ground as far forward as possible.

Now the chin is drawn back followed by the nose, until nose and forehead once more touch the ground as they did in the beginning.

It will save you much time if you study the above carefully in detail and so acquire the correct technique.

Repeat three times, with a pause at the end.

Advice to beginners: To ensure that the arms play *no* part, you may either raise the palms slightly one or two centimetres from the ground or put the hands behind your back, the left one holding the right.

The final motionless stage of the asana follows the third active ascension.

Now a complete reversal takes place: the arms, which until now have not been taking part, are to become the *sole* active muscle element, while the back remains passive. This is usually forgotten, and the effectiveness of the posture is reduced in consequence.

From now on, the arms alone are used to bend the spinal column back. If the movement is to be perfect, the back and legs must take absolutely no part. It is a good idea to pause before the arms take the strain, so that the back is first given time to relax.

While this stage is in progress the adept should be able to feel in the nape of the neck the pressure and the bending which spreads from vertebra to vertebra down to the lumbar and sacral regions of the spinal column. Do not forget to relax the buttocks, thighs and calves. At this stage the feet tend to separate a little: they should be left to position themselves correctly.

The flushing in the back moves down to the base of the spine (into the kidneys and sacrum). (See 'effects on the kidneys and adrenal glands', p. 148 etc.)

It is *very important*, at this point, to ensure that the navel is kept very close to the ground.

Another common mistake which reduces the good effects of the posture is to allow the neck to drop awkwardly between the shoulders. The head should be held proudly and the shoulders level, which means that the curvature increases to reach its maximum, the arms being still slightly bent and the elbows held in to the body. If, in the final position, the arms are tense and straight, it means that the hands were not properly sited at the start, or it could be that the stomach is being raised too much or, possibly, that the shoulders are not being lowered properly.

VARIANT ON THE FINAL POSITION

The final position having been reached then, either: the head is kept straight, the eyes looking forward (see photograph, p. 152) or the eyes look towards the ceiling, and the head is tilted backwards as far as possible (see photograph, p. 152).

The latter variant is the more correct of the two, but since it acts upon the thyroid gland, it is not quite so suitable in cases of hyperthyroidism.

A. Within a series of asanas

In the final stages the pause lasts for three to ten breaths made as deep as possible. Start with three and add an extra one each week.

B. When practised as an isolated posture

If, however, the posture is practised by itself and for its own sake, immobility may be sustained until you feel tired. The asana may be repeated several times, with a rest period between each. The total duration here may be several minutes.

FOR BEGINNERS

At the outset, if you are unable to raise the head much, do not attach too great an importance to the failure. So long as your technique is correct, you will still benefit from the exercise, as you can see from the flushing in your back, which will occur at the first attempt, providing the instructions given above are followed.

BREATHING

Breathe normally throughout, stopping only if your personal teacher says otherwise. You have only to perform the asana once with restricted breathing for the face instantly to become over-congested –a very undesirable effect. If the breath is held, it is tiring. For yoga done properly should never lead to fatigue, but should leave one overflowing with energy and high spirits. In the static period, the breathing will deviate a little from the normal: it is, however, necessary at this stage to breathe as deeply as possible, otherwise breathing is reduced through the stretching of the abdomen.

CONCENTRATION

Should be focused on the movement during the dynamic stage. Think of the pressure set up and spreading along the spine, vertebra by vertebra.

During the static stage, concentrate on the spinal column as a whole.

CONTRA-INDICATIONS

There are virtually none, so long as the asana is practised correctly, without violent or jerky movements. If you feel pain at any stage, you should reduce the amount of effort you were using. Be gentle with yourself–there is no need to put up with discomfort or pain!

At first the back may be slightly painful and stiff, but this should disappear within a few days.

The posture, if it is to be really effective, must not be practised too energetically at first. The flushing in the back, which you will be able to see at the first attempt, shows that the bloodstream is not irrigating in depth the muscles of the spinal column–the life-axis of the body.

FAULTS

Guard against any of the following:

—at the beginning of the posture, placing the hands in an exaggerated forward or backward position;

—pushing with the arms during the dynamic stage;

—straightening the arms completely (even at the end of the position they are never quite tensed);

—separating the elbows from the body (they must be kept close to the sides);

—opening the mouth;

—bending the knees;

—raising, rather than lowering, the shoulders;

—raising the navel too high from the ground (it should be as close to the floor as possible).

EFFECTS AND ADVANTAGES

The good effects of the Cobra come from the magnificent backward bend of the spine, and the substantial strength given to the muscle structure of the grooves of the spine.

During the active stage the strain is taken by the abdomen, so that the internal pressures are increased. During the static stage, the stomach is stretched. In both cases the entire viscera are toned up. This asana warms up the body.

Spinal Column

Flexibility = youthfulness.

This incomparable asana induces suppleness in the spine, which is the source of health, vitality and youthfulness. A sedentary life, with

146

its lack of movement, stiffens the spine: worse still, bending over our work we set up more or less pronounced cyphoses, with which Bhujaṅgāsana effectively contends. If the curvature of the spine is very pronounced—which it often is—the adept will find it difficult to master the posture. He should not be deterred, for Bhujaṅgāṣana is a real blessing.

The Nervous System
The atrophied dorsal and vertebral muscles which are so widespread in our civilization, are responsible for a mass of unfortunate symptoms, above all because they reduce the flow of blood round the spinal cord, on which the circulation in the muscles lying round the vertebrae depends. It is vital for these muscles to be exercised daily and Bhujaṅgāsana is excellent in this respect. There is no need to dwell on the essential importance of the spinal cord: the whole activity of the nervous system passes, at any given moment, by way of the vertebral column, which is bordered by the two chains of ganglia belonging to the sympathetic nervous system, whose activity also reaches into every organ of the body. If these nerves, ganglia and other vital structures, receive the abundant supply of blood, which is their due, the health of the organism is ensured. If, however, the supply of blood is insufficient, the organs depending on these nerves deteriorate in time and disorders arise, resulting in various types of organic lesion.

During the period of immobilisation, the flow of blood to the lumbar and sacral regions stimulates the pelvic portion of the vagus nerve—and corrects the balance in the ortho-sympathetic ganglia.

The Endocrine Glands
The action of the thyroid gland is normalised, if there has been any slight departure from the normal. Pathological cases such as goitre, etc. must receive medical treatment. Bhujaṅgāsana also tones up the supra-renal medulla, which manufactures adrenalin, the hormone which promotes energy. A healthy supra-renal gland also means that a normal production of cortisone is being maintained, which guards against certain forms of rheumatism.

Alimentary Canal and Accessory Glands

The posture has a favourable effect on the digestive system as a whole, because it alternately compresses and stretches the abdomen. Bhujaṅgāsana fights constipation. During the static period and deep respirations, the liver, gall-bladder, spleen and pancreas are stimulated by the gentle and deep massage.

The increase in intra-abdominal pressure acts on the kidneys while the posture is held; the blood is forced from the kidneys, and during the return to the starting position they receive a valuable supply of fresh blood, which cleanses them and helps diuretic activity.

The Thoracic Cage

The increased suppleness of the spinal column, above all the correction of cyphoses, lessens the rigidity of the chest, which expands.

Effects on the Health

This posture combats constipation, genito-urinary disturbances (amenorrhoea, dismenorrhoea, leucorrhoea), and regularizes the menstrual cycle. It allays flatulence after meals.

A sedentary life immodilises us in abnormal positions and leads to various troubles, especially in the small of the back, so that it becomes painful to stand erect. The Cobra posture is the best and surest remedy, because it exercises the spinal column. There are instances where small stones in the gall bladder have been evacuated through the cystic duct as a result of practising the Cobra.

Some forms of sciatica are improved – even cured – by it, although in certain cases the posture can accentuate the pain, because if the vertebrae are displaced, the sciatic nerve becomes compressed. Pain is always a sign that one has attempted too much. If the method is followed carefully, there should never be any pain. Nevertheless if pain does arise, all that is necessary is to practise more gently or to cut short the exercise, when you will once more revert to your normal state.

Aesthetic Effects

A round back is as ugly as an emaciated one. You will no longer be ashamed to show off your prominent vertebrae in a decolleté gown or two piece suit, because Bhujaṅgāsana will develop the dorsal muscles and hide the vertebrae without making you look like a prizefighter. A good muscle structure gives a marvellous shape to a feminine – and a masculine – back!

Psychological Effects
A rounded back and hunched shoulders give a sense of insecurity and inferiority. On the other hand, an upright carriage makes you worthy to be a human being: the supple spinal column, with its muscular support, gives you self-confidence, whether in a bathing-suit or wearing your best clothes.

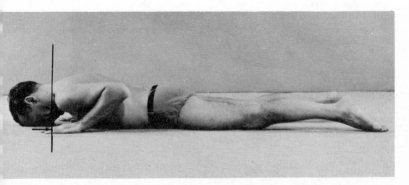

FAULT The hands are not in the correct position and the legs are parted.

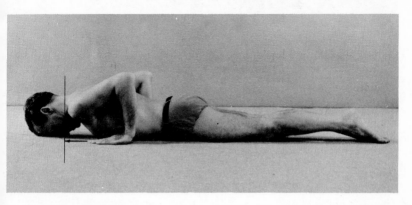

FAULT The mistake lies in the position of the hands, which this time have been placed too far back.

149

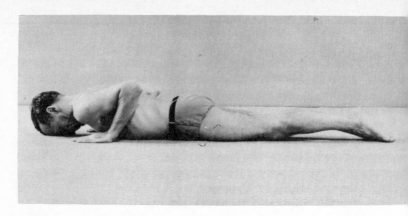

Correct starting position. Notice particularly the position of the hands in relation to the shoulders. The elbows are close to the body, feet together, and knees as well. Relax for a moment before beginning the movement.

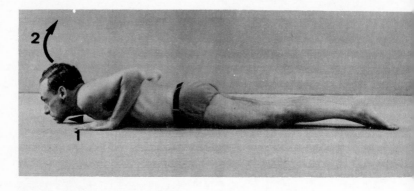

First Part of the dynamic stage.
The chin is pushed forward as far as possible, and touches the ground. A feeling of tension in the neck proves that the movement is correct.

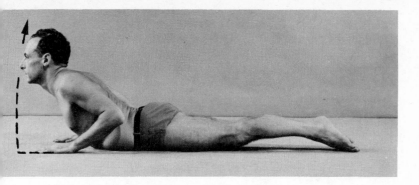

Second Part of the dynamic stage.
By pulling on the muscles of the nape of the neck and the back, the body
is *very* slowly raised.
The arms do not take part in the movement, but are totally relaxed. Keep
the legs together.

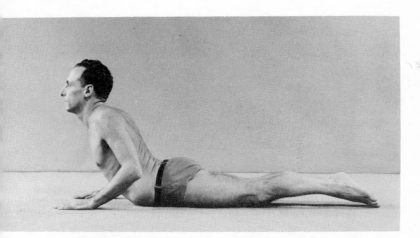

End of the dynamic stage.
The muscular structure in the back is contracted to its fullest extent so as
to raise the trunk as high as possible. Arms and hands still remain non-
active and relaxed.

The pressure in the abdomen reaches a very high level, and the back
flushes considerably. The legs are stretched out and held together.
Return to the ground and repeat this movement three times more.

151

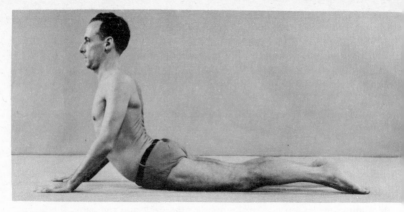

At the end of the third movement, we pass on to the static stage, in which the arms are used to push the back as far up as possible. The back remains inactive; so do the legs, which means that the feet are slightly parted. Remain motionless and breathe deeply from three to ten times.

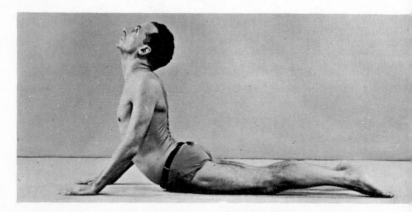

The above variant, which some yogis prefer, differs in the head position alone. The nape of the neck is stretched slightly, and the neck is compressed; both these factors contribute to the effectiveness of the posture.

This variant is a more comprehensive one. Those with any condition of hyperthyroidism are advised to practise the previous posture instead.

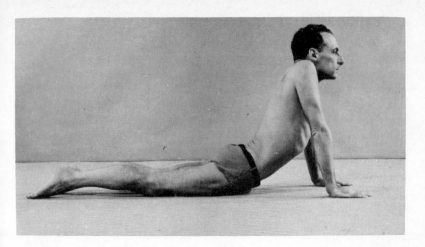

FAULT

This photograph illustrates two very common errors.

—the elbows have been raised instead of being properly lowered.

—the stomach fails to touch the ground. It should be kept as close as possible to the floor.

These faulty positions may deprive the posture of a great deal of its good effects, reducing the curvature, as well as the pressure in the loins, almost to nothing.

21. *Shalabhāsana: The Locust*

Shalabha in Sanskrit means a locust.

METHOD

There are varying degrees of ever increasing difficulty in this asana. Ardha-Shalabhāsana or the Half-Locust is followed by the complete Locust, and finally one or other of the more advanced variants.

Unlike the Cobra, the Plough and Forward Bend, etc., Shalabhāsana is an almost entirely active exercise. The static stage is therefore very short.

Ardha-Shalabhāsana: The Half-Locust

Starting Point

This asana follows and completes the Cobra. The starting position is almost identical in both cases. The adept is therefore lying flat, face downwards, legs stretched out side by side, with the soles of the feet turned up as in the Cobra, but the arm and head positions are slightly different, the arms being placed at the sides of the body, palms flat on the ground. It is essential throughout the exercise to keep the whole length of the arms from shoulder to finger-tips, touching the floor.

Place the chin on the floor, pushing it as far forward as possible. This will stretch the neck, and simultaneously compress the nape. A large proportion of the benefits stems from the activity in the nape of the neck. (see 'Effects', p. 159).

CARRYING OUT THE ASANA

Introductory note

This asana is very easy, so that anyone can perform it: briefly it consists of raising the right and left leg one after the other as high as possible . . . although not just anyhow!

Before you begin you must realize that, in Ardha-Shalabhāsana, at first *only the left half of the body* is put to work, while the other half is kept as relaxed as possible. Now alternate the movement. Thus, when the left leg is raised you must lean on the left arm, contracting only the muscles in the left side: work in the opposite manner when raising the right leg.

During Ardha-Shalabhāsana the pelvis should neither twist nor rise to any extent.

Now we are ready to proceed! Slowly raise the left leg by contracting the muscles in the small of the back, lean on the left arm, although at this stage the weight of the legs is largely transferred to the abdominal region where the pressure increases. Do not:
—bend the leg
—tense the calves
—point the toes violently.

The foot should rise perpendicular to its former position on the floor. Cheating a little by tilting the pelvis, and putting the weight on the opposite knee, you will be able to raise the leg much higher than if you follow the description given above. This is by the way. You must keep to the essential which is the *contraction* of the muscles in the lower part of the back, which brings a plentiful flow of fresh blood to the lumbar region, thus completing the effects of the Cobra. Pause, then bring the leg back to the floor. To assess how much is lost by doing the exercise wrongly, practise it both ways and you soon find out.

Usually if you do Ardha-Shalabhāsana twice in succession–that is by raising first the left then the right leg, and repeating the whole movement you are ready for the full Locust.

The Complete Locust
METHOD
Starting Position
The initial position is identical in all but one detail to that of Ardha-Shalabhāsana: the fists must be clenched to provide more strength.

In the complete Locust both legs are raised simultaneously by a strong contraction of the muscles in the small of the back.

Be careful to avoid bending the knees, stiffening the calves or pointing the toes like a ballet-dancer.

Here, even more than in the Half-Locust, it is essential to keep

155

the shoulders and chin in contact with the ground throughout the movement. At the beginning it does not matter if the shoulders rise; you can do your best to bring them as near to the floor as you can: a little patient practice and you will get it right. Keep the legs up for a few seconds then bring them gently to the floor.

Some yogis turn the palms up – a minor detail. Try both ways and choose the one you prefer.

VARIANT 1

'Why have the yogis named this exercise "the Locust posture" since it has no resemblance to that insect?' Variant No. 1 provides the answer: the folded arms resemble the legs of the insect. When you are quite at home in the normal asana, you will have no difficulty with this variant.
Note that:
—the hand is not placed flat on the floor; the palm forms an arch, and most of the pushing is done with the finger-tips – the shoulders do not leave the floor.

VARIANT 2 (for advanced students)

Although in its first stages Shalabhāsana is within the scope of everyone, the final yogic phase is one of the hardest in yoga, since it requires the greatest flexibility in the lumbar region, together with a powerful back. In its final form it is, to our knowledge, the only yogic exercise which allows – and indeed requires – a thrusting movement.

Starting Position
This differs from the preceding ones in two details:
—the chin is not pushed as far forward as possible, instead the nose touches the carpet.
—the fingers are entwined, the arms brought towards each other, and placed under the thorax. In the photograph it is easy to see the special hand and arm positions.

Taking up the Asana
The whole weight of the body rests on the chest and arms. Breathe in deeply, hold the breath, and with one sustained effort, raise the legs to the vertical position.

We have just suggested that the breath should be held, but this is valid only in the second variant.

In all the other forms of Shalabhāsana you must *breathe normally throughout*. This is more difficult in the Locust than in the other yogic exercises. You must however persist, and leave breath retention techniques to advanced adepts.

CONCENTRATION

The adept must concentrate upon every muscle in action, particularly on those in the base of the back (lumbar region and *lattissimus dorsi*).

DURATION

Shalabhāsana takes up very little time:

Ardha-Shalabhāsana includes a pause of a few seconds at the moment when the feet are at their highest point, nothing more.

A pause of from two to five seconds in the final position is generally enough.

In the second variant it is rarely possible to hold the position for more than ten seconds.

There is a short relaxation period after Shalabhāsana. Wait until the breathing has returned to normal, before passing on to the next posture in your series.

The complete exercise may be repeated from two to five times.

IMPORTANT

Even advanced adepts should move daily through every stage in the Locust posture: that is, through the half-Locust, complete Locust, and occasionally the advanced variant, because each one prepares the body for the next, and produces different effects.

HELPFUL EFFECTS

A brief run through our knowledge of anatomy and physiology becomes essential, if we are to understand what the good effects are. Remember that all involuntary activity in the body, both conscious and unconscious, is controlled by the autonomous nervous system, which is divided into two separate and opposite systems, one acting as an accelerator, the other slowing down the activity. The balance of these two activities provides for the proper working of the ultra-

157

complex machine which is man, and hence for his health and span of life. It consists of:

(a) the *sympathetic* system, which is made up of a double chain of ganglia linked together by a network of nerves, lying parallel to each other on each side of the spinal column;

(b) the *para-sympathetic,* its opposite number, itself divided into two parts:

(i) the pneumogastric or vagus nerve, linked with the medulla, the bulbous section lying between the skull and the spinal cord, and emerging from the spinal column at the point where it supports the skull. It innervates the heart and lungs, the stomach, and a large number of other visceral organs, before losing itself in the complex of nerves known as the solar plexus.

(ii) The sacral portion of the para-sympathetic system which branches from the spinal column in the lumbar region, to innervate the pelvic viscera, including the genital organs.

These two portions work as a whole, and in harmony. It is therefore essential to stimulate them and tone them up in a balanced manner.

The Locust is invaluable because it tones up the sacral portion of the para-sympathetic system by drawing blood into the base of the spine through the powerful contractions in the muscles there.

What is more, since the head and shoulders are kept on the floor throughout, the asana acts on the neck and nape, particularly at the point where the vagus nerve branches from the spinal column. That is why the shoulders must stay on the ground, while the chin is pushed as far forward as possible.

In addition, every point that we made about the Cobra applies, in almost every detail, to the Locust which complements it.

Finally, the viscera are toned up through the increase of intra-abdominal pressure.

The effects described in detail above proceed from these factors.

Spinal Column
The posture increases its flexibility, especially in the lumbar region.

Muscles
The lumbar muscle formation is strengthened considerably; this

is invaluable, because lack of exercise resulting from a sedentary life threatens most civilized people with larval atrophy in these muscles, which may lead to a displacement of vertebrae, particularly near the fifth lumbar vertebra, on which the whole spinal structure rests.

We shall be saved from any number of disorders if we can strengthen the muscles in this region. How many acute attacks of lumbago, 'backache', are caused by weak muscles and ligaments in this part of the back! The slightest jolt or false movement may bring on a variety of dislocations, some of which – sciatica for instance – are highly disagreeable. We should add in passing a word about chairs – so often a danger to this region of the back because the shape of the seat and back of the chair is all wrong – a well-muscled and supple back is not at risk, but this is not true of the back which suffers from civilization.

The situation is so alarming that every year one American in seven suffers from back trouble, which, in the USA, has become the primary factor in wastage of industrial manpower. Even President Kennedy was forced to wear a special corset to support the back. Is it not better, then to reinforce the dorsal muscles?

The housewife is subject to the same risks, and often a faulty working position is to blame: ironing for too long at too low a board for instance, or cooking at a stove that is too low.

A spinal column which is not based on sufficient muscular strength is at risk if it lifts even a medium amount of weight. Shalabhāsana is not the only asana designed to strengthen the spinal column, but it is certainly one of the very best to protect it against accident.

The Nerves
The Locust recharges the centres of the nervous system, particularly those which control the lower part of the stomach, as well as the solar plexus.

The Alimentary Tract
This exercise has a powerful effect on the kidneys by reason of its deep internal 'massage', which favours diuretic action.

The digestive system as a whole, and its accessory glands, are massaged, toned up and stimulated.

The Locust considerably improves the functions of the liver and pancreas, and regularizes the workings of the intestines so that peristaltic action increases.

The Circulation of the Blood
Raising the legs benefits the circulation of the blood, and here Shalabhāsana rounds off the effects of the inverted postures. First of all, the excess venous blood is forced from the veins in the legs, so that varicose veins are prevented. Then, since the arterial blood has to fight the force of gravity if it is to reach the feet, it irrigates the lower part of the stomach and sacral region where the influx of blood is further increased by the muscular contraction.

The Lungs
In more advanced adepts, who have progressed to breath retention, the air pressure increases in the lungs during this asana. The lungs are strengthened since this pressure acts upon the alveoli, to unfold them, improving oxygenation, and ensuring an improved fixation of oxygen.

Aesthetic Value
If the faulty curvature in the back of the spinal column can be corrected, then the whole deportment is favourably influenced.

OCCULT EFFECTS
The practice of this asana produces occult results, through the awakening of Kundalini, but all this lies outside the scope of this book.

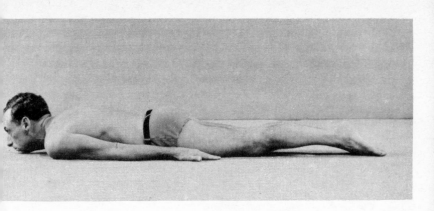

The legs are together, and the shoulders touch the floor. Pay particular attention to the position of the head, which is very important.

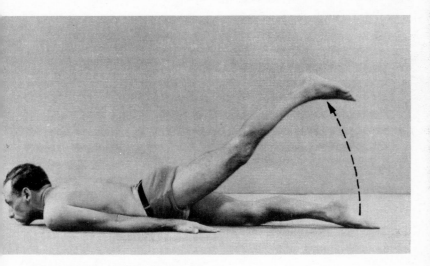

Ardha-Shalabhāsana (*Half-Locust*)
Slowly raise each leg in turn. The movement is initiated entirely by the muscles in the lower back. The pelvis does not turn, the knees are not bent, and calves are relaxed.
Repeat at least twice.

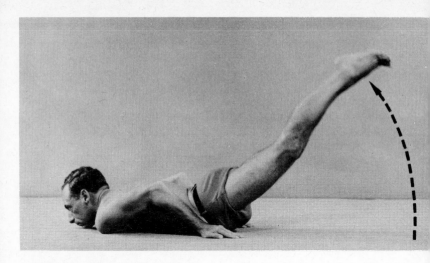

Complete Locust (*Variant* 2)
The position of the arms differs from that in the last exercise. The propulsion comes from the finger tips as the palms are arched.
As before the chin and shoulders remain on the ground throughout.

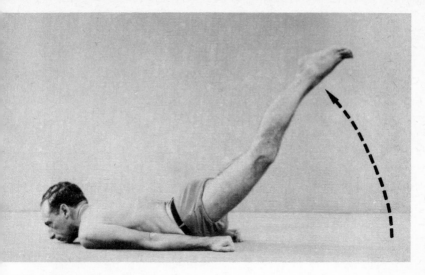

Shalabhāsana (*Complete Locust*)

Both hips are raised by contracting the muscles in the base of the back. Pause from one to five seconds before returning to the ground. The fists are clenched. The movement may be repeated from three to five times if desired. Breathe normally, The chin does not rise and the shoulders remain on the floor. The knees do not bend but stay close together.

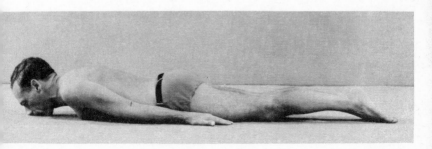

FAULT
Incorrect starting position.
The chin is not pushed forward and the elbows do not touch the floor.

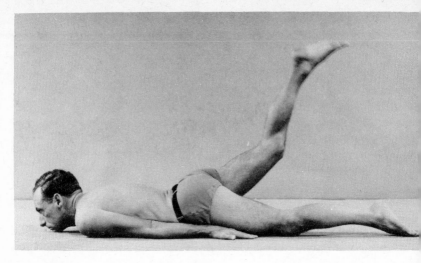

FAULT
The head position is correct and the elbows touch the floor, but the leg is bent, and is not raised exactly above the place where it lay at the start. The pelvis is slightly tilted—another fault.

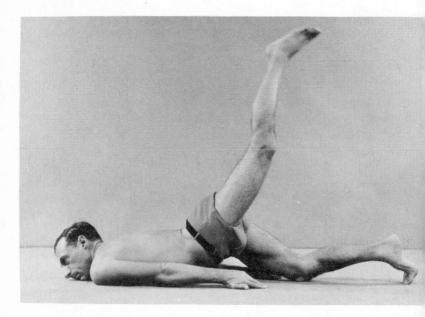

FAULT
In this demonstration almost every possible mistake is being made! The head is wrongly positioned. The shoulders touch the ground which is correct, but the leg is supported by the pressure of the other knee on the ground. The pelvis has left the floor and is twisted. Try this out and you will realize that it has practically no effect at all.

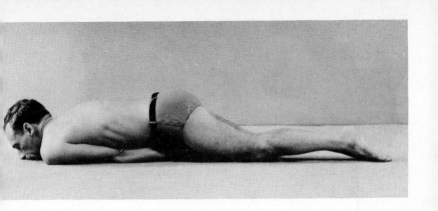

ELABORATED VARIANT (for advanced adepts)

Starting position
Note the position of the chin. The hands are clasped, wrists nearly together. Their exact position is not visible in this photograph but may be clearly seen in the following one:

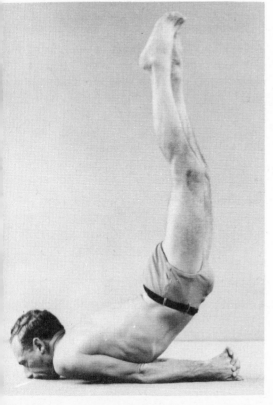

Carrying out the movement
Breathe in and hold the breath. By means of a powerful contraction, raise the legs and pelvic region, bringing the legs up to the vertical. The shoulders must stay as close as possible to the ground. This is a fairly difficult exercise and should not be undertaken until after long experience of the normal Locust posture.

165

22. *Dhanurāsana:*
The Bow

This posture gets its name from the bending of the body, like a bow.

The Bow – a great classic in yoga, combines unequalled effectiveness with simplicity – by no means the same as 'easiness'. Indeed, for the beginner it is one of the most awkward of the asanas: he may well think of it as a 'hard' exercise, to be tamed by force and violence. This is wrong, since not only is it possible, but also essential, to practise it without undue effort. The Locust and the Cobra, are the ideal preparation for the Bow.

Since the Bow is a combination of the Cobra and the Locust, it is not irrelevant to wonder whether they duplicate each other. But they do not, because although Dhanurāsana completes the other two, it differs widely from them: in the Cobra and the Locust, the muscles of the back are *active,* in the Bow they should remain *passive.* Dhanurāsana includes a second stage which is little known and rarely taught in the West, but which should nevertheless be learnt. Its performance only adds a few seconds to the session.

STARTING POSITION

Dhanurāsana is practised after the Locust. The adept lies flat on his stomach with his arms alongside the body.

The position of the head and the direction of the palms are of little importance. Above all see that the back is totally relaxed, because it is on this that the success of the exercise depends.

FIRST PHASE

Raise the chin, simultaneously grasping the ankles with the hands. Beginners may hold first the right and then the left ankle. The photograph on p. 172 shows the exact placing of the hands and fingers. Notice the position of the thumb, which is in line with the fingers.

The legs are the *only* propelling factor in Dhanurāsana. Even the arms remain passive, as they merely link ankles to shoulders like a cable, while the fingers grip with just enough force to maintain their hold.

To carry out the asana, the feet must be pushed back and up by a powerful contraction of the thighs and calves, which raises the shoulders and arches the back. Therefore, apart from the legs and fingers, the rest of your body should remain relaxed throughout: if for instance, the back is tensed, the asana becomes impossible.

At the beginning the knees often remain despairingly stuck to the floor and if they do succeed in rising a little, it is only at the cost of some pain in the thigh muscles. Be patient! In the final position the knees should rise above the chin. In fact, the bend in the knee should be level with the top of the skull (position A), and not, as in position B, where the knees are only level with the chin. In the latter position the weight of the body is borne partly by the iliac crest, thus decreasing the effectiveness of the asana. In the position A, when the knees are brought above chin-level, the pubis does not touch the ground, and the body's weight is borne by the pit of the stomach, which increases pressure on the viscera, so producing the maximum effect.

DYNAMIC STAGE: ROCKING

The dynamic stage begins as soon as the asana has been taken up and consists in making rocking movements like those of a rocking chair or horse.

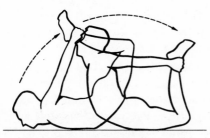

MAXIMUM RANGE OF THE
ROCKING MOVEMENT

At first the movement is slight and limited to the abdomen, but it gradually increases, passing from the chest and the stomach, until the thighs touch the ground. It gives a *very* effective and powerful abdominal massage.

We scarcely need to point out that, during all this, it is impossible to keep the back completely relaxed.

DURATION OF THE DYNAMIC STAGE
This clearly depends upon individual ability: you should not continue until you become breathless: usually four to twelve rocking movements will do. It is less trying if you do two or three movements and then return to the start for a short period of relaxation.

BREATHING DURING THE DYNAMIC PERIOD
There are three alternatives for breathing at this stage:

(a) inhale when the head rises; exhale when it drops;
(b) breathe normally;
(c) hold the breath with the lungs full: this is reserved for advanced adepts.

CONCENTRATION
During the rocking movements you may concentrate either on the back or the abdominal muscles.

STATIC STAGE
This consists in immobilizing your body in the full posture, without undue strain, either before or after the dynamic stage: try out both, adopting the one you find most comfortable.

BREATHING AND DURATION
During the static stage breathe normally. Trained adepts will now take a series of deep breaths, which are held as long as possible without discomfort. This increases the intra-abdominal pressure still further. Generally speaking, five to ten respirations are a good average. Dhirendra Bramachari, who was *guru* to the late Mr Nehru, used to advise: 'Hold as long as you can' (within the limits of comfort).

168

If the adept has been concentrating on the abdominal massage while rocking to and fro, he should now focus his mind on the back so as to relax it deeply.

RETURN

Reduce the leg-thrusts, and return *slowly* to the starting position. Relax and wait until the breathing becomes normal, before passing on to the next exercise:

FURTHER DETAILS

Position of the Knees:

While Dhanurāsana is being performed, the knees may be kept apart, and this helps the exercise without reducing its usefulness, provided that the big toes are touching throughout, failing which the feet will nearly always be at different levels owing to the slight deviations present in every backbone. If a conscious effort is made to keep the big toes together, then the whole spinal column works within its perfect axis, and faults in the posture of the spine will be corrected.

Position of the Chin:

We have already made clear the respective positions of chin and knees, but the distance of the chin from the floor is also important: it should be raised as little as possible, so that the weight falls on the pit of the stomach.

EFFECTS

The Bow, since it combines the Cobra and Locust, adds their advantages (see the description of the effects of those two asanas) to its own, which are derived from the increase of the intra-abdominal pressure to tone up all the viscera, especially when deep breathing accompanies the exercise, the diaphragm exerting a powerful massage on every organ.

Spinal Column

As in the Cobra and the Locust, the compression of the dorsal part of the rachis, and the stretching of the anterior surfaces act upon the ligaments, muscles and nerve centres in the spinal column. The Bow prevents untimely calcification in the vertebrae, and straightens backs hunched through years of sitting at desks, in offices or at work-benches.

Muscles

At the start, pain is felt in the thighs, and, if it is true that painful yoga is yoga badly done, then this muscular pain is mild; in any case, with practice it decreases and soon disappears.

The stretching of the muscles in the abdominal region helps with Uḍḍiyāna Bandha, the abdominal squeeze.

The feeling of 'freedom' and the euphoria given by this asana, stem from the stimulation of the nervous centres in the spine, and especially of the sympathetic nervous system.

Let us also list the forceful effects upon the solar plexus, the complex of nerves lying in the pit of the stomach – the place 'below the belt' so dreaded in the boxing ring. The rocking movements massage and stimulate it gently and effectively.

We know how anxiety can make the stomach lurch disagreeably, through congestion in the solar plexus' region, which exerts a negative influence over the autonomous functions and leads to a variety of functional disorders, which do not yield to current treatments. The rocking and stretching of the abdominal muscles, in addition to the massage produced by deep breathing from the diaphragm, dispel these symptoms.

Cellulitis and Overweight

Dhanurāsana combats cellulitis, the causes of which are: insufficient respiration; general nervous tension; poor assimilation of food; and reduced circulation in the cellulitic patches.

The Bow posture helps by: increasing the breathing; decongestion of the solar plexus; and improving the circulation in the cellulitic or fat masses by gentle and regular massage.

The Endocrine Glands

The Bow acts on the suprarenal glands: the increased secretion of adrenalin increases energy in those inclined to lassitude, at the same time guarding against over-stimulation. The secretion of cortisone is regulated and this helps to combat various forms of rheumatism.

170

Autogenous cortisone has none of the ill effects of the chemical variety, which is administered by injection in the treatment of certain illnesses.

The pancreas resumes its normal function, manufacturing the insulin so essential to the metabolism of glucagon.

Cases of false diabetes brought on by anxiety (there is, for example, a temporary degree of diabetes mellitus in soldiers at the battle front and in students during examinations) disappear completely in a very short time. This is due to decongestion in the solar plexus and normalization of the pancreatic function induced by the practice of this posture.

According to Swami Shivananda, the Bow posture also acts on the thyroid gland.

Alimentary Canal and Accessory Glands

The increase in intra-abdominal pressure works upon the whole digestive apparatus and its accessory glands. Dhanurāsana helps to decongest the liver, which is massaged by it, especially during deep respiration and increases the circulation of blood throughout the digestive system. Do not, therefore, undertake the exercise on a full stomach. The Bow contends with constipation by improving peristaltic action in the intestines.

The kidneys are well irrigated and are greatly benefited by Dhanurāsana, which helps them to eliminate toxins.

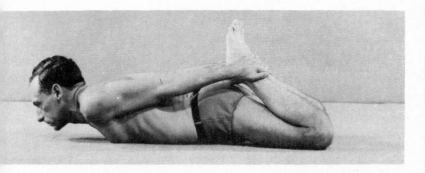

Starting position: Take hold of the ankles simultaneously with both hands. Notice the position of the fingers and particularly of the thumbs. The chin is raised slightly off the floor, the knees are parted but the toes touch! Breathe normally.

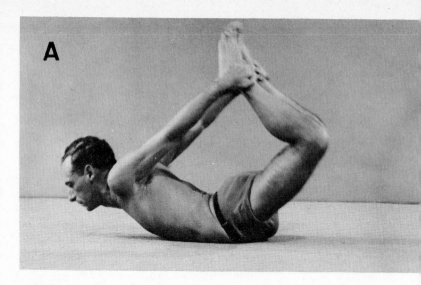

A

Push the feet back and *up*. The knees are raised higher than the chin, even above the top of the skull; the pubis therefore leaves the ground. The weight of the body rests on the pit of the stomach. The arms are sufficiently tensed (muscles relaxed) to ensure that the ankles and shoulders are linked. They are not bent. The back relaxes. Do not frown. The knees are apart but *the big toes held together*. Breathe deeply so as to increase massage in the abdomen.

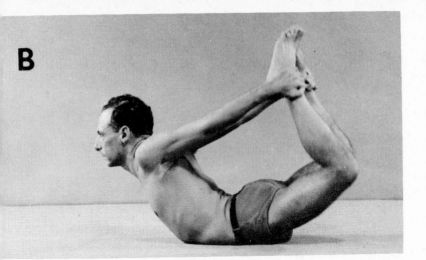

B

This position is not incorrect. It differs from the previous one, only in so far as the pelvis now carries some of the weight of the body, because the chin is raised higher than the knees, so that the pubis does not leave the floor. The intra-abdominal pressure, therefore, is less than in the asana illustrated in the previous photograph. This is desirable in some cases.

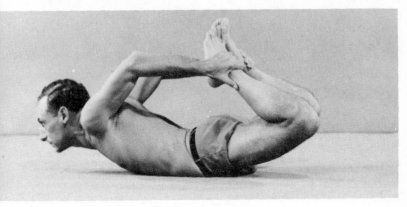

FAULT

The following mistakes appear in this photograph:
—the feet are grasped too high;
—the toes do not touch;
—the arms are working instead of being relaxed;
—the back is tensed.

These factors lead to an insufficient arching of the back. The effort is violent, but the results are meagre.

173

ADDITIONAL STAGE
to be carried out after the Bow Posture

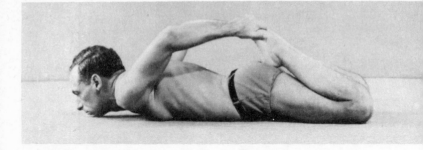

Initial position
The hands grasp the feet as high up as possible, thumbs turned upwards. The heels are applied to the buttocks and remain in this position throughout the exercise. The chin touches the floor and remains in contact with it throughout. The arms prepare for the movement. The legs are *relaxed*.

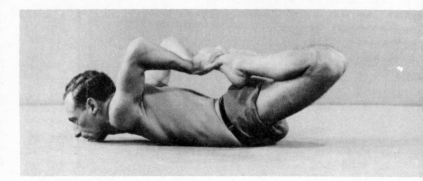

Final posture
By pulling on the back muscles, and by thrusting with the abdominal muscles, knees and pubis both leave the ground. The feet still touch the buttocks and the chin rests on the ground. Breathing is normal; the legs relaxed and inactive. The arms act as the moving force. In this exercise the muscles which were relaced in the classic version of the Bow are now tensed, and vice-versa. This position is negative to the other.

23. Ardha—Matsyendrāsana: The Twist

This asana which is undoubtedly the most plastic and aesthetic of all is one of the few called after its inventor – the great Rishi Matsyendra. The original posture is however, very difficult and inaccessible to any but the most accomplished yogis and so we shall teach the half (Ardha) posture; which we shall call by its Sanskrit name, although you will often find it described as the *twist*, *twisted* or *spinal* posture.

GENERAL REMARKS

While the other asanas bend the vertebral column, Ardha-Matsyendrāsana *twists* it throughout its length.

This exercise should feature in every series of asanas since it concludes the successive forward and backward bends.

It is individual from the first, since it starts from the sitting position rather than from the recumbent, and contains no dynamic stage.

METHOD

Fortunately the asana is easier to perform than to describe.

VARIANT FOR PRELIMINARY WORK

We suggest that beginners should first practise the variant as a preliminary; anyone can do it and it produces the same good effects as the complete asana. Here it is:

Starting Position

Sit on the floor, legs extended in front of you, feet together. Double up the *right leg* (an important detail!) and place the foot against the outside surface of the left knee, with the external malleolus, or ankle-bone touching that knee. The right foot is flat on the ground, parallel with the left leg.

Now, place the *left* arm against the knee of the bent right leg. Normally the armpit should rest on the knee, but this is not always possible for the beginner.

TAKING UP THE ASANA

With the arm serving as lever, bring the left hand up to the extended left leg and try to touch the shin, or, if possible, grasp the right foot. The spinal column is further twisted by a thrust from the right arm placed behind the back, the hand pressing on the floor. The twist moves from the sacrum step by step up the spine until, by turning the head, it reaches the nape of the neck.

Slowly return to the starting point in the opposite direction, and practise the posture on the other side, that is to say by bending the left leg.

During the twisting, the line of the shoulders remains as far as possible parallel to the floor.

Classic Position

After a short time the adept will be able to move on with ease to the classic posture, which differs from the preparatory one in the following details:
—the leg, which was stretched out is now bent, to bring the heel against the thigh.
—the arm, which was pressed against the floor behind the back, now encircles the waist, and the hand tries to touch the thigh.

In the final position the back is held very erect so as to accentuate the twist.

IMPORTANT

Throughout the asana the back remains *passive:* the arms induce the shoulders to turn, and the spine twists without offering any resistance. Do not rotate the pelvis, but remain seated on both buttocks throughout. The slow and progressive turning is carried out while the breath is being exhaled. The head turns at the last moment, remaining very straight, with the chin held fairly high.

Hold the following position:

—the heel of the bent leg touches the perineum, the knee remaining on the floor;
—both thighs touch the carpet;
—the line of the shoulders is horizontal;
—the fingers grasp the foot under the *arch* of the sole;
—the knee is almost in the armpit;
—the hand of the arm encircling the waist moves towards the groin and touches the thigh;
—the head is straight, the eyes fixed as far as possible to the rear.

We have stressed how essential it is to double up the *right* leg first: that is to say the right thigh is pressed against the abdomen, so that the colon is compressed. In the description of the beneficial results obtained from this asana, you will see how it increases peristaltic action in the intestines, diminishing constipation – the 'curse of the century'. It is to follow the proper peristaltic movement that the right side of the abdominal region is compressed first.

CONCENTRATION

Concentrate on relaxing the muscle structure in the spinal column, and follow mentally the progression of the twist as it moves from the sacrum to the skull.

DURATION AND RESPIRATION

This posture is not normally repeated, when assumed in a series of asanas. The immobile period from five to ten breaths on each side. These should be as complete as possible so that the massage of the viscera is intensified by the pressure of the thigh upon it.

Only advanced adepts are able to hold the breath with the lungs filled while the posture is being maintained.

As in every yogic posture Ardha-Matsyendrāsana may also be practised on its own, so as to distil from it the maximum benefit.

In this case it should be maintained severely motionless for not more than three minutes on each side, that is six minutes in all.

BENEFICIAL EFFECTS

The benefits of this asana result from:

(1) the twisting of the vertebral column;
(2) the alternate compression of each half of the abdominal region.

Effects upon the Vertebral Column
(a) *Muscles and ligaments.* The twisting movement stretches and lengthens every muscle and ligament in the spinal column, where it produces a considerable flow of blood, so that the back is flushed. Ardha-Matsyendrāsana tones up the muscles in the vertebral column, prevents or removes soreness in the muscles of the spine, and engenders an immediate sensation of well-being.
(b) *The Nerves.* Considering how important the vertebral column is with its spinal cord and chains of sympathetic ganglia on either side, it is not difficult to understand how this asana tones up the organism, and also why yogis regard it as a powerful factor in the process of rejuvenation.
(c) *The Vertebral column.* This is what Kernéiz says of it:
  'The main object of this asana is to avoid the sacralisation of the fifth lumbar vertebra, that is, to prevent its becoming fused with the sacrum, or, rather, to guard against this condition before it begins to set in.

  This immobilisation happens so frequently, that those suffering from it usually look upon it as normal, and allow it to develop without even attempting to guard against it, until it has become an acute infirmity characteristic of old age. It is not often nowadays, that we manage to keep our normal ability for walking after the age of fifty. The extreme degree of contraction which results from this ankylosis, gradually gains ground in our minds so that we settle into the sorrowful and crabbed humour which is a typical feature of old age.
(d) *The Endocrine glands.* Ardha-Matsyendrāsana has a benign action on the suprarenal glands.
Abdomen
Ardha-Matsyendrāsana tones up all the viscera by compressing each half of the stomach in turn. The colon is involved to an important degree and its peristaltic activity is stepped up. We must repeat once again that it is essential always to begin by compressing the *right side of the stomach*, in order to work with the direction of the peristalsis. This is how the asana helps in removing constipation Apart from the large intestine, the liver and the right kidney are stimulated during the first half of the exercise, and the spleen, pancreas, and left kidney during the second half.

These derive from the reasons already stated. Ardha-Matsyendrāsana:

—tones up the sympathetic nervous system and revives the organism;
—corrects deviation in the spinal column;
—prevents lumbago, 'backstrain', and even certain forms of sciatica;
—helps in the process of diuresis by stimulating the kidneys, and the suprarenal glands;
—combats constipation, stimulates and decongests the liver and the whole of the alimentary canal;
—combats obesity and cellulitis in the stomach.

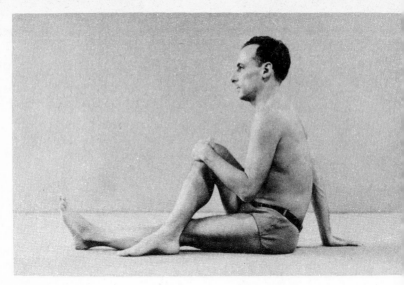

In a sitting position, first bend the *right* leg, and place the right foot against the outsi surface of the left knee.

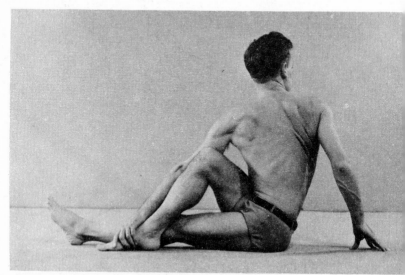

Leaning with the left arm pushed as high as possible to the shoulder, and against th right knee, prise the arm up so as to twist the spine, and now grasp either the shi or right foot as shown in the photograph. Push with the left arm, hand on the floo behind the back. Turn your head right round.

One detail is *wrong*: the external ankle-bone is not positioned exactly against th bend of the knee. The foot being placed too far ahead, the line of the shoulders doe not run parallel with the ground.

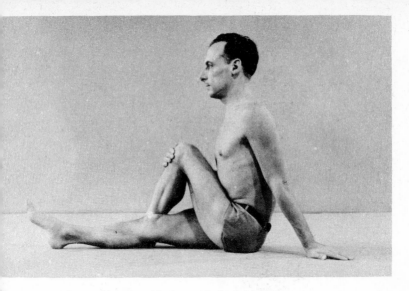

The same starting position, but this time with the *left* leg bent up.

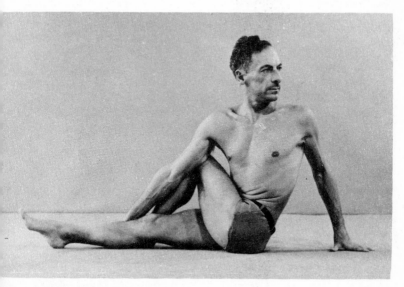

Final position of variant for beginners.

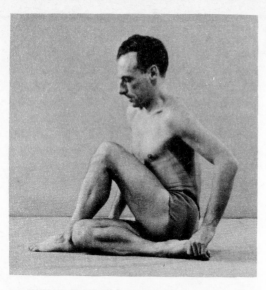

Starting point of the clas
Ardha-Matsyendrāsana.
left leg is folded, and the h
placed against the perineum.

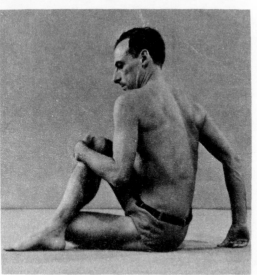

Starting point of Ard
Matsyendrāsana seen from
other side, to demonstrate
bent leg, with the heel rest
against the perineum.
knee must touch the ground

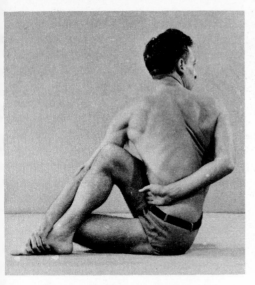

Final posture, seen from the back, showing position of the right arm, and of the hand which should be touching the thigh. This demonstrates the correct way to grasp the foot.

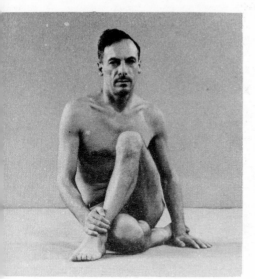

The same seen from the front.

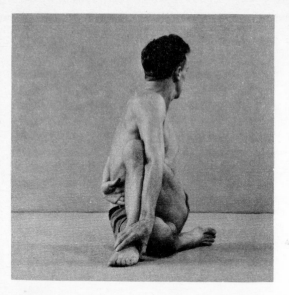

Seen in profile, showing the position of the foot, which is flat on the ground, and parallel to the leg, which in its turn is brought up against the body. The knee touches the ground. Sit as straight as possible so as to "untwist" to the maximum extent.

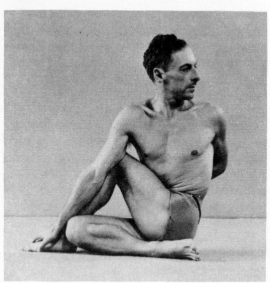

Final posture of Ardha Matsyendrāsana in it classic form; it is unquestionably aesthetic.

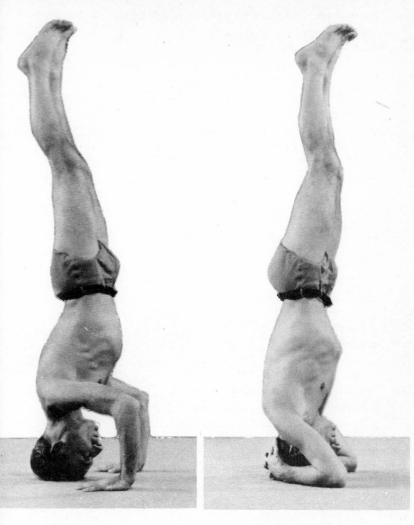

Kapâlâsana   **Shirshâsana**

24. *Shīrṣāsana and Kapālāsana*

In yogic literature the headstand is known by a variety of names: 'Shīrṣāsana' is the most usual, and 'Kapālāsana' is another.

The posture represented in the photograph and described in the following pages is the classic one. 'Shīrṣāsana', while Kapālāsana (from the Sanskrit Kapāla = cranium), illustrated in the second photograph, is the 'tripod' posture – more easily accessible to beginners.

METHOD

You must persuade yourself from the first that Kapālāsana is neither an acrobatic turn nor a feat of strength. Its most difficult feature lies in taking up the position from a correct departure point, and then holding it for a few seconds at the beginning, gradually increasing the time, in order to strengthen the neck and the nape of the neck, and to condition the brain to receive the increased flow of blood.

Notice that the preliminary posture – although to a lesser extent – in itself produces all the effects provided by Shīrṣāsana.

Be sure to place the head and hands correctly on the floor. If it is too hard, you can use a blanket folded in four; this is better than a cushion which is too thick and soft, and therefore unstable.

25. Shīrsāsana: The Head-Stand

Shīrṣāsana—the head-stand—is beyond doubt the best-known of all yogic postures, so much so that the public tends to speak of 'yoga' and of 'standing on one's head' in the same breath. Does it owe its fame to its very oddness? Or is it because yogis think of it as the queen of the asanas? No matter!

To those who are not adepts, it seems madness to perform head-stands; 'What on earth for, I might break my neck!–Besides it's very bad to allow the blood to run to the head!'

Beginners in the West, especially the younger ones, are attracted by the spectacular character and beneficial effects of Shīrsāsana, while apprehensive of its acrobatic side, which they feel, has its dangers.

We consider that if only one asana could be practised it would have to be Shīrṣāsana.

Why stand on the head when we have so much trouble in learning to balance on our feet, so that our first steps marked one of the greatest days in our lives?

Man is the only being to hold himself upright; an attribute unique to him, and a fatal one at that, because man *became* a human being when he acquired it. We rose up from the earth and our forelegs turned into hands, which are really extensions of the brain. Set free and able to grasp objects, the hand of man has become a creative tool, the only one by which he may crystallize his thoughts. This creative activity in its turn has forced man to use his brain in resolving his problems–and so it was that, gradually evolving, both hand and brain developed together in mutual sympathy. When we look at evolution in perspective, the upright position is seen as a relatively recent achievement–an adaptation still imperfect, above all as it affects the spinal column and the circulation of the blood.

In the quadruped (the horse or dog for example), the bulk of the body remains parallel to the ground, and gravity acts evenly on it, so that the circulation, working horizontally, is not much influenced by it. In man, on the other hand, the circulation operates in the vertical plane, and gravity exerts an overwhelming influence upon it.

Below the heart, it is the venous circulation which is mainly affected. To reach the heart and lungs, the venous blood must overcome the force of gravity, relying on muscular contractions which compress the veins and force the blood up, the valves preventing any backward flow. This solution was satisfactory in natural man, who was forced to expend muscular energy in order to survive, but the muscular contractions in sedentary civilized man are insufficient to ensure an adequate rate of venous circulation. As a result, the venous blood accumulates in the legs and still more in the stomach; it stagnates in the viscera, and impairs their proper function. Man in his natural state breathes deeply and fully, thanks to the piston-like movements of the diaphragm. The blood is stirred up, and there is a powerful intake of venous blood into the lungs which (like sponges), soak it up as well as air with every inspiration. The deeper the inspiration, the greater the quantity of blood to enter the lungs. Breathing and circulation therefore work directly together.

This part played by the lungs as a suction-pump for venous blood, is quite insufficient in sedentary man, whose breathing is superficial.

In those parts of the body which lie above the heart, the return of venous blood is helped by the force of gravity; but, on the other hand, the arterial circulation is slowed down, above all in the neighbourhood of the brain: and this is even more disastrous to the civilized being, who is almost entirely a cerebral creature, and whose brain, greedily consuming oxygen, is bound to require an extra allowance of blood!

It is not only the circulation which suffers from the erect position. In animals, the abdominal organs remain in place and do not prolapse. In man the vertical position is responsible for 'floating kidney', prolapsus of the stomach, dropped intestines, and so on; all are sources of grave functional disorders.

This is the logical reason why yogis recommend the head-stand, to eliminate, instantly and infallibly, the disadvantages which stem from standing upright.

EFFECTS OF THE HEAD-STAND
So numerous and varied are the effects of the queen of asanas, that

we cannot describe them all. Let us look at the main ones, without getting lost in a maze of detail; for the essential thing is to know where and how the results are procured.

EFFECTS ON THE SKELETON

We shall first look at its effect on the carriage of the spinal column. In countries where women carry water in heavy pitchers on their heads, it is noticeable that the vertebral column is perfect, the bearing graceful and supple. The ability to carry a load balanced on the head indicates that the skull and the neck are held in a position which must affect the whole spinal column.

In training to be models, girls acquire a graceful carriage by carrying first one book on their heads, and then increasing the number gradually.

Shīrṣāsana produces these results automatically and in accentuated form, because in this exercise the whole weight of the body rests on the skull.

The action extends also into the base of the spine, particularly into the articulation of the fifth lumbar vertebra and the sacrum, which supports the whole weight of the human body, except for the legs. The disc is especially liable to damage, because it is subjected to the maximum amount of pressure. Just think what strain it is forced at times to stand – when riding a horse for example. In quadrupeds the sacrum is scarcely more than the junction between the pelvis and the spinal column; it has no weight to carry.

In Shīrṣāsana the lumbar vertebrae have to support only the weight of the legs and pelvic girdle. When a perfectly-balanced head-stand is achieved, the lumbar vertebrae are automatically placed in their normal and, incidentally, their most favourable, position. This is why Shirṣāsana banishes, in a matter of seconds, that 'backache' which is caused by prolonged hours of standing.

It is true that the cervical region receives the whole weight of the body, but this does not endanger the nape of the neck in any way, providing it is normal; more especially because the nape has been settled into a defensive position, that is to say it has subsided onto the shoulders. A child at play will sometimes grasp the nape of your neck from behind, whereupon the head is instinctively placed in a position to render it least vulnerable.

But it is the circulation which derives the greatest benefit from the head-stand. We know that standing upright increases stasis in the veins which lie below the level of the heart, owing to the gravitational pull, while above the heart it is the arterial blood supply which is retarded.

Shīrṣāsana reverses the situation: the venous blood, now helped by gravity, is at once evacuated from the legs, while blood stases are eliminated from the abdominal organs. The massed venous blood in the legs is recirculated and its return to the heart is speeded up. The volume of arterial blood in circulation, then, depends on that of the venous blood, because the heart is a force-pump—nourished with the blood which has been purified and oxygenated by the lungs. Since the return of venous blood is stepped up, the lungs receive an extra supply to be purged of toxins. The head-stand, therefore, when combined with deep breathing, cleanses the organism without tiring the heart, which beats purposefully and calmly.

The arterial blood pours in quantity, and under gentle pressure, into the brain, whereas if the subject is standing upright it is forced to fight against gravity to get there. (See 'Effects upon the brain' p. 192).

The veins of the legs are more rested than they can be in the recumbent position. Shīrṣāsana prevents varicose veins and haemorrhoids; if you are predisposed to them, this posture will help to prevent them becoming more acute, and will gradually rid you of them altogether.

In this case it is a good idea to complement the action by spraying the affected parts with cold water, in addition to any treatment which may have been recommended by your doctor.

EFFECTS ON THE ABDOMINAL REGION

The stomach is the factory, the workshop, of the body, and the region between the diaphragm and pelvic girdle is of vital importance.

Apart from reactivating the circulation of stagnating blood in the abdomen, Shīrṣāsana also decongests the viscera in the lower stomach region where a condition of more or less permanent congestion is created by prolonged sitting.

In passing, we should note that the prostate troubles which beset so many men after the age of fifty, are aggravated – if not caused – by this congestion. In the head-stand the prostate gland is cleared, and an immediate improvement is felt.

The genital organs are likewise freed of congestion. Any prolapsed organs (the kidneys, stomach, or intestines) resume their normal place and shape with progressive and systematic practice, which will enable you to hold the position long enough to achieve curative results (some three to five minutes, say an average total of a quarter of an hour daily).

One of the principal organs to feel the benefit of Shīrṣāsana, is the digestive tract and its accessory glands, notably the liver which, in so many people who lead a sedentary life, may suffer from larvated congestion. If we remember that all the venous blood in the digestive system passes through the liver, we can at once understand the importance of avoiding any hepatic congestion. Here too the venous circulation conditions the arterial circulation and *not the reverse*. If the venous blood is drained from the digestive system, an influx of arterial blood will enter, and with it an improvement in digestive function.

During the head-stand the liver enjoys a useful degree of massage; it is an organ which is very easily compressed, and will flatten against the diaphragm, that semi-cartilaginous, semi-muscular wall, which separates the abdominal organs and the lungs within the thoracic cage. In Shīrṣāsana, if the subject is breathing deeply, the up and down movement of the diaphragm massages the liver together with the whole weight of the viscera resting on it. The spleen which is often congested benefits as well from this massage, although to a lesser extent than the liver.

THE LUNGS

The head-stand produces a fundamental difference in the method of breathing. Whether we are sitting or standing, the lungs are sited at a higher level, which, when the position is reversed, becomes the lower.

We have just made it clear that the abdominal organs exert pressure on the diaphragm: when we hold the breath, the air in the lungs will be under slight pressure; and this will cause the pulmonary alveoli to unfold harmoniously, favouring the passage of oxygen through the pulmonary membrane, without hindering to any degree the evacuation of carbon dioxide which, thanks to its physical properties, can very easily escape.

191

Shīrṣāsana is particularly effective during exhalation, the fundamental stage in breathing. Incomplete exhalation implies the permanent stagnation of the vitiated and toxic residual air in the lungs, and this reduces the quantity of air breathed in, since no receptacle can take in more than has been emptied from it! How many poor pairs of lungs in civilized men are as badly ventilated as their owners' homes!

Shīrṣāsana facilitates deep exhalation through the pressure of the organs on the diaphragm. That is why yogis affirm that this posture leads automatically to pranayama, providing you *breathe through the nose*.

A final point which is basic for our health: in this posture the apex of the lungs is well aerated, and this prevents tuberculosis; for Koch's bacillus, the recognized cause of this disease, dies when brought into contact with the oxygen in air. If everyone breathed deeply, sanatoria would be wiped out, or turned into Yoga centres!

EFFECTS ON THE BRAIN

Before we speak of the effects of Shīrṣāsana on the brain, we shall look at some figures. The brain–that gigantic ant-heap where billions of nerve cells live and work–is the most highly vascularized organ in the whole body, because the amount of blood it requires in comparison with the needs of other organs and tissues is enormous. The brain is daily irrigated by an average 2,000 litres of blood: I repeat *two thousand!* As you know, the capillaries are minute blood vessels through which the red corpuscles circulate. But did you know that their total length adds up to 100,000 kilometres? (see Doctor Salmanoff's *Secrets and Wisdom of the Body*.) Did you know, too, that one gramme of muscular tissue contains about eight metres of capillaries; one gramme of cerebral white matter, three hundred metres, the cerebral cortex, the well-known 'grey matter', one thousand metres! Just think: a kilometre of living blood-vessels to each gramme. These capillaries are elastic, and very sensitive to variations in pressure. Distended and slack they allow the corpuscles to pass too easily. Clenched and in spasm they become obstructed. During Shīrṣāsana, the blood, assisted by the force of gravity, increases in quantity, and under light pressure (harmless except in cases where the contra-indications described on pp. 194 and 196 exist) rinses the network of blood vessels in the brain.

Shīrṣāsana conserves or restores the elasticity of the capillaries. The plentiful rinsing and opening up of the cerebral capillaries in their state of spasm, does away with most forms of headache and migraine,[1] often as though by magic, without recourse to drugs.

Shīrsāsana promotes and stimulates the intellectual functions. It improves both memory and concentration, and increases resistance to nervous fatigue. Many states of anxiety and neurosis disappear when the exercise is practised daily. Obviously it cannot turn an idiot into a genius, but the improvement in the function of cerebral physiology gives everyone the chance to develop his intellectual resources to the full.

The skull also shelters the hypophysis, or pituitary gland–tiny, measuring no more than a centimetre, weighing six grammes, and buried in the warm depths of the head. There also lies the hypothalamus, which orchestrates the action of all the other endocrine glands, affecting the entire organism. Shīrsāsana regularizes their function, together with that of the thyroid, which above all controls the metabolism, and contributes greatly to keeping the organism young. Removing the thyroid from an animal leads to rapid ageing and premature death, while pathological changes in that organ cause cretinism.

Shīrṣāsana also helps us to preserve or restore our normal weight; it will assist those who should reduce to lose weight, while those who are underweight will find themselves gaining.

THE SENSORY ORGANS

Sight

Shīrsāsana has surprising effects on the sensory organs. The eyesight can be *seen* to improve–the analogy is apt–because the ocular system in general (including the cerebral centres of vision), and the retina in particular, great consumers of oxygen, benefit largely from the strong supplementary flow of arterial blood. To convince yourself of all this, before you start the exercise place one of those reading cards used by opticians, or a newspaper, at a distance of six feet, and then quietly look at its whole surface without straining your eyes. Now stand on your head, shut your eyes for a minute, and look again. You will find that you are already seeing more distinctly.

[1] Do not confuse 'migraine', which only affects one half of the head, with 'headache' which involves the whole.

Contra-Indications

Those who are threatened with detachment of the retina should not do this asana. The same applies to any eye defects which are really diseases, such as conjunctivitis, glaucoma, etc. On the other hand myopia, presbyopia, and astigmatism, which are all connected with slight deformation of the eyes, whether temporary or not, escape this proviso. What is more, Shīrṣāsana can do them nothing but good.

Hearing

The hearing can also be improved by the practice of Shīrṣāsana.

Contra-Indications

Those suffering from otitis and other inflammatory infections of the ear should not do the head-stand until some time after they have been cured.

The Cerebellum

The cerebellum is an organ the size of a small tangerine, situated at the base of the brain. Linked with all the voluntary motor centres, it is concerned with co-ordinating the body's movements. If an animal is deprived of its cerebellum it remains alive and conscious, but becomes awkward, its movements clumsy and ill-co-ordinated; it can scarcely keep its balance. The cerebellum plays a special part in carrying out balanced movements – of which Shīrṣāsana is one.

AESTHETIC EFFECTS

In improving the deportment of the vertebral column, Shīrṣāsana rewards us with a straight, natural posture, and a graceful, supple carriage. The skin of the face receives such a plentiful supply of arterial blood, that it is better nourished than by any anti-wrinkle creams. Lines show first on the forehead, and at the corners of the eyes near the temple (crows' feet), because these are the least well irrigated areas. But with the practice of Shīrṣāsana the skin grows younger and is regenerated, incipient wrinkles are ironed out (except for the deep furrows which are engraved on the brow), the complexion freshens, and the whole face reflects well being. Yoga tradition has it that the hair will grow again if the scalp is well supplied with blood, so essential if baldness is to be treated. Greying hair will begin to regain its colour after a year of this exercise. However if you are to achieve this regeneration you will have to practise Shīrsāsana daily for at least half an hour, which, if necessary, may be divided into several sessions.

Shīrsāsana produces many other effects which it would be tedious to list in detail. Let us content ourselves with the main ones and . . . with practise the asana will produce results, including some we have not mentioned. And this is all that matters.

We have only one thing to add, and that is to say how greatly Shīrsāsana assists in overcoming insomnia, and improves the circulation of blood to the feet! Indeed after you have held the posture for a few minutes, and then returned to your normal position, you will see how pink and warm your feet have become.

CONTRA-INDICATIONS

The contra-indications to the head-stand are less severe and numerous than might be feared, while experience has proved that cases to whom it must be strictly forbidden are rare. It can be mastered by ninety per cent of those who practise it progressively.

Although we ourselves have taught hundreds of people – some of them over sixty years of age – we have not recorded a single instance of unfortunate consequences from this asana. It is all a question of proportion and common sense. The methods indicated in this book eliminate those who might be harmed by this posture.

Obviously if there is sclerosis of the arteries and arterioles of the brain, then it should not be undertaken. The same is true in cases of marked hypertension and aneurysm. Although even here the danger is minimal, since sufficiently clear warning signs are soon apparent.

Should the head-stand immediately bring on a violent attack of migraine which becomes more acute at each fresh attempt, then you should give it up, at least for the time being.

If there is buzzing in the ears, increasing with every practice, care must be exercised. To start with, there may well be singing or humming in the ears, but this will gradually decrease, is normal and should give no cause for anxiety. High blood pressure becomes a contra-indicator if the arterial tension falls below 9. Slight giddiness may sometimes be felt, but this is harmless, and often due to the sudden return to an upright position after the practice.

In *every case* one or the other of the two positions illustrated on page 202 must be taken up immediately after the posture, so that the circulation can revert to normal.

IMPORTANT!

If Shīrṣāsana is performed wrongly it can produce a feeling of suffocation, the consequence of a violent effort to achieve the posture or an unconscious obstruction of the breath. Never, therefore, use force, but continue to breathe normally through the nose while doing it.

At first avoid any risk by keeping to the initial exercises. They will accustom you to being upside down, and will strengthen the neck muscles. They prepare the vascular system of the brain for the gentle pressure caused by the influx of blood.

While you are carrying out these exercises, your legs do not rise to the vertical position, and since the pressure is in proportion to the level of liquid in a column (shades of physics lessons!), this remains constantly within the safe limit.

AGAINST THE WALL OR IN THE MIDDLE OF THE ROOM?

In the initial stages for beginners, the wall is a doubtful ally because it provides artificial support which sometimes induces them to go beyond their capabilities. Only after mastering the initial exercises in the middle of the room, (you cannot fall – at the worst you may collapse gently), can you go on to propping yourself up against the wall, and so to a fully upright position.

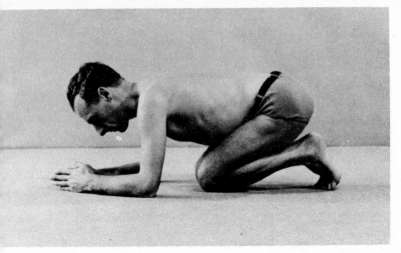

For a correct starting position, place the head at the apex of an equilateral triangle, and the hands at its base. Use your elbows to determine the sides of the triangle.

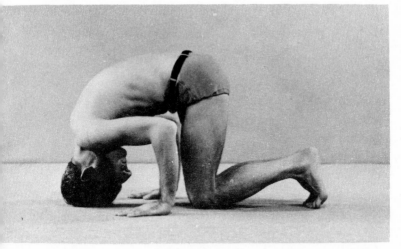

Head and hands have been placed at the angles of the triangle referred to above; now the skull must be placed correctly on the ground. The weight of the body is to be borne at a point near to the front of the cranium. This is *very important* because the way in which the head is placed on the ground conditions the deportment of the spinal column while the complete posture is being held. If the resting point is too far to the back, the back itself will be curved when you attempt to stand on your head, and you will collapse . . . not that you will come to any harm, but you will not have succeeded in your exercise.

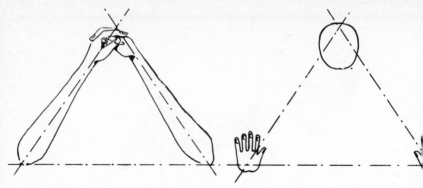

Determine the triangle   Correct position for head and hands

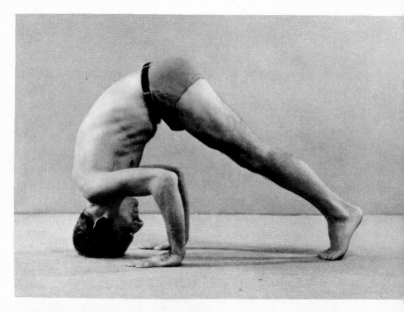

When the head and hands are correctly placed on the floor, straighten the legs, thus transferring some of the weight of the trunk to the skull. You will see from the photograph above that the position of the head in relation to the floor, has not changed.

Throughout the exercise, the final position included, the skull will continue to rest at the same point on the floor, and the head will remain as if screwed into the floor. At first, older people, or those whose necks are too fragile, should not hold this position for longer than a few seconds.

They will gradually extend the time, as and when the neck muscles become stronger. When you feel that your neck is strong enough to support more weight . . .

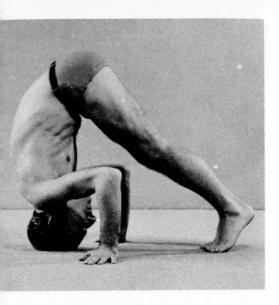

Some people prefer to place their hands differently; as, for example, in this photograph. It is perfectly permissable, but they must be kept at the same angle throughout the exercise.

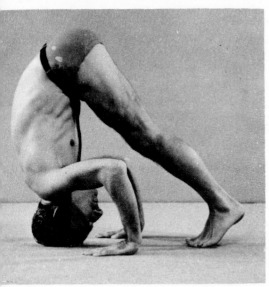

. . . still keeping the legs tensed, bring the toes closer to the head. Almost the whole weight of the trunk is now resting on the skull.

199

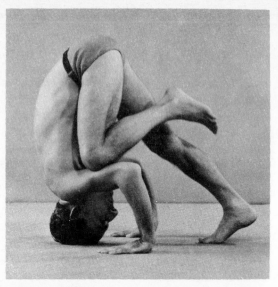

When you have brought the toes as close as possible to the head, without in any way displacing the position of the skull on the floor bend up one leg and place it on the arm, a few centimetres behind the elbow, the foot pointing inwards.

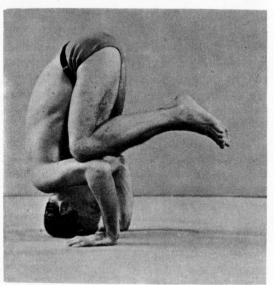

In the same way place the other knee on its corresponding arm. According to individual capability, these various stages may stretch over several consecutive days or weeks of training, or they may take only a few minutes, and be reached at the first attempt; but it is always better to attempt less than your potential. When you can keep this position with ease, then the head-stand is 80 per cent achieved and the total posture presents no further difficulties.

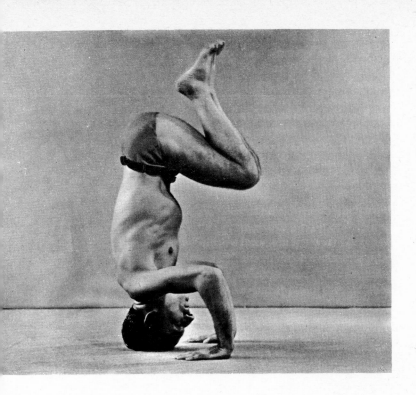

Begin by bringing the feet as close as possible to the thighs, so as to raise the whole body in a curled position. Then by contraction of the muscles in the base of the back (lumbar region), lift the knees a little from their resting-place on the elbows. At the start you will only manage to raise a few centimetres—then when you can feel that the movement is going to be made from the hips, rise higher. Keep the weight of the body consistently on the same point of the skull. Settle the increased weight in a backward direction, this may cause you to collapse, but this is nothing to worry about; should you feel yourself overbalancing, bring the knees up against the chest and you will simply roll over on to the floor: when you are ready for it, you should practise this overbalancing movement, by bringing the stomach towards the inside of the triangle which is formed by the top of your skull, with your palms applied to the floor, and then hollowing the back.

If you carry out the exercise in the middle of the room, be careful to see that there is no furniture in the way, in case you do overbalance.

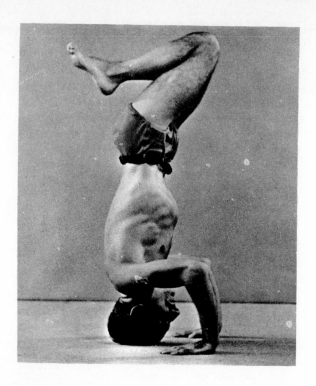

Once you have succeeded in raising the knees as far as the horizontal position, continue the movement, lifting them further, and pointing them up, at the same time keeping the feet as close as possible to the thighs. Do be careful not to make the mistake which has been mentioned elsewhere of raising the legs too soon, without first having brought the feet in against the thighs, in which case your final position would be incorrect.

When the knees are pointing correctly up, unbend the legs and you will automatically find yourself in the correct position. Now it is only a question of finding, through gradual practice, the zero point, that is to say, the perfect balancing point in which the head can remain without further muscular effort and in which you are able to relax. In the perfected headstand, every muscle in the legs, back, abdomen, and biceps, is relaxed.

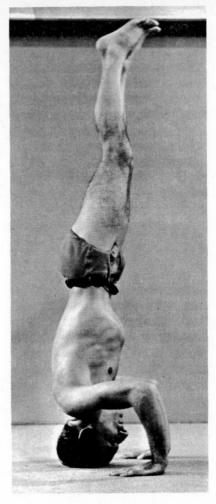

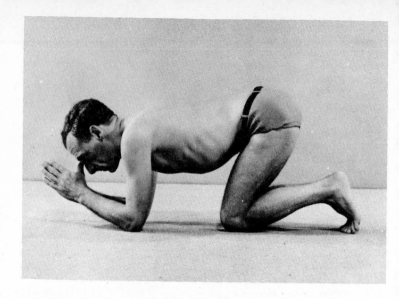

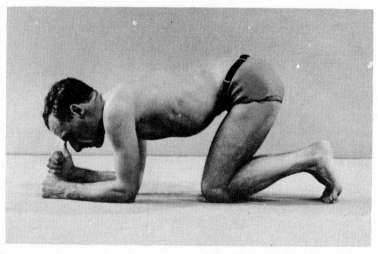

When you have done the head-stand, or even after you have exercised in the preparatory positions, it is essential to take up one or other of the two positions above (they are of equal value; the choice is one of personal convenience), so as to restore normal circulation.

This remark is addressed, not only to beginners, but to all who practise the head-stand in one form or another.

The thumbs are placed against the arch of the brows, so as to allow the neck to relax. This position should be held for from fifteen to thirty seconds.

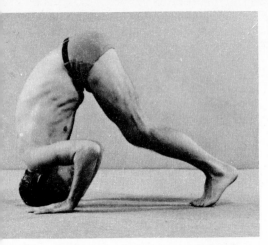

AVOID THE FOLLOWING MISTAKES

FAULT

The hands are incorrectly placed on the ground. They are too close to the skull and the base of the triangle is too small; it is difficult to balance securely, and you will be unable to assume the complete posture.

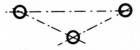

FAULT

Nor should the hands be placed too far behind, which is just as bad. The triangle is larger, but the abnormal position of the forearms will not permit the hands to be placed flat on the floor —an essential factor, if the starting base is to be firm enough.

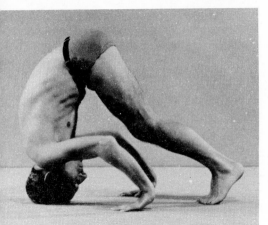

FAULT

This photograph illustrates a mistake which is very widespread; the knees are not applied to the arms. but lie alongside. This makes it very difficult to raise the legs in order to assume the final posture.

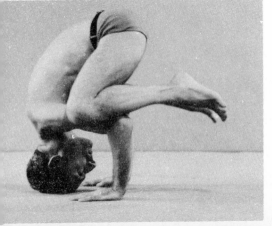

205

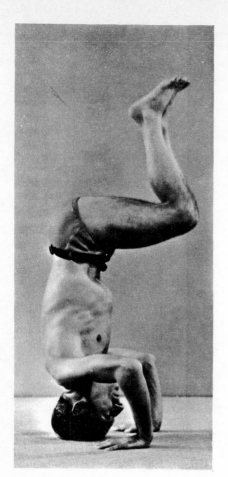

In addition to the most frequent mistakes made in practice of this posture, that of failing to take the weight of the body on the same place in the skull, which may make you overbalance backwards, two more mistakes are illustrated here: the feet, before they were raised, have not been brought up against the thighs or the knees pointed towards the ceiling.

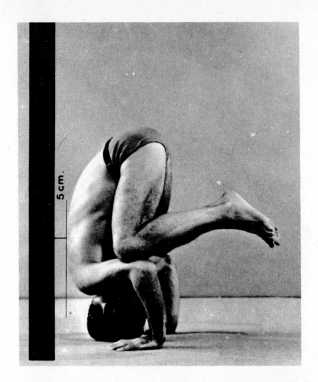

5 cm.

If you are afraid of falling you may exercise near a wall, which when you are in the starting position, should be 5 centimetres from your back. If nearer it will prevent you from raising your body properly; if further away, it becomes a danger instead of a precaution, since you risk a fall by bending your neck against the wall. Although not dangerous, you could wrench a muscle, which is not pleasant.

Once you are able to hold this starting position comfortably, Kapālāsana no longer presents any major difficulty.

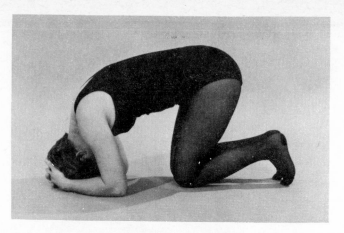

Now that you have mastered Kapālāsana, you will very soon be capable of taking up the head-stand in the classic Shīrṣāsana.
The start for most people is more difficult than for Kapālāsana, but the final position is more comfortable, which is why yogis prefer it.

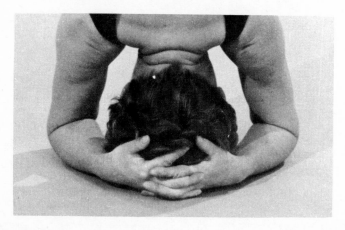

Entwine the finger loosely. Fold the elbows as shown in the photograph. The fingers do not come to rest beneath the skull but rather against its dome where they act more or less as a prop, but do not really provide much support. The fingers should prevent the head from rolling about and should keep it in the starting position, so that it never moves at any time during the exercise.

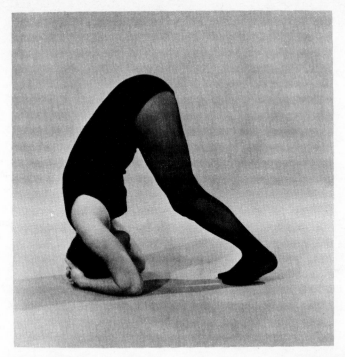

Straighten the legs and bring the toes in towards the face. The body's weight still rests on the same part of the skull. Place the maximum weight on the head to lighten the work of the arms.

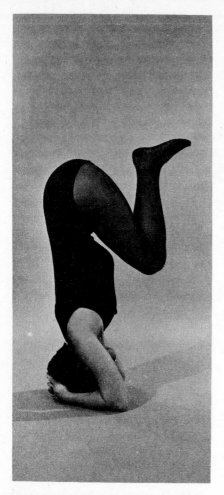 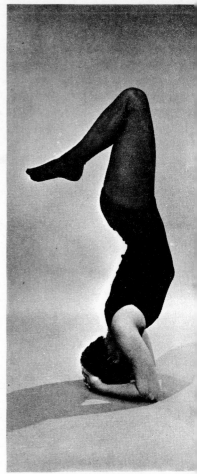

When you can bring the feet no closer to the face without tipping over backwards, bend the legs and bring the feet up against the thighs.

To raise yourself up, proceed as for Kapālāsana. Point the knees towards the ceiling before raising the feet.

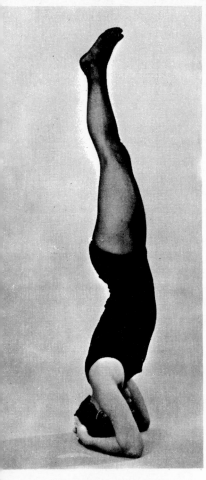

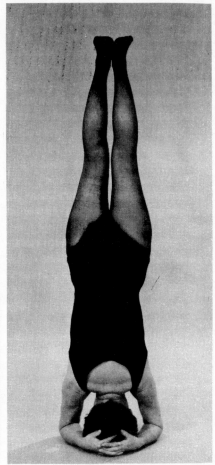

Now carefully look for the zero point, concentrating your whole mind upon relaxing the muscles, from the toes up to the neck and the nape.

Make sure the nape of the neck is settled correctly, then bring the shoulders down as low as you can, failing which you will tire easily.

26. *Uḍḍīyāna Bandha*

How ought we to translate Uḍḍīyāna Bandha? 'Bandha' in this context means 'blockage, contraction', and 'Uḍḍīyāna' is made up from the Sanskrit roots 'ut' and 'di', meaning 'to fly upwards'. This does not really enlighten us much, and neither does the yogic assertion that the exercise causes 'Prana to fly upwards by the Sushumna Nadi'.[1] We shall bypass the problem by using the Sanskrit name.

INTRODUCTION
The abdominal exercises are distinctive and spectacular, and the sight of an adept pulling in his entire abdominal region makes a great impression on the uninitiated.

Yet Uḍḍīyāna Bandha is not difficult! In Hatha-yoga it is as easy as the floating position is in swimming, and once the mechanics are understood even the first attempt has a great chance of success. A Bedouin who has never seen a man swim, would scarcely believe his eyes could he see a man floating. By the same token you cannot know much about yoga if Uḍḍīyāna makes you feel like Koestler, when he wrote: 'He [the yogi] began with the classic exercises, such as uddiyama [*sic*] drawing in the abdominal muscles, while forcing the viscerae and diaphragm upwards, until a large, hollow cavity appears under the ribs, a kind of incredible grotto in the flesh, and the *obliqui abdomini*, the two transversal muscles, stick out in a rather horrifying manner as on anatomical figures stripped of skin . . . It was fascinating and faintly nauseating to watch . . .'

Koestler was unfortunate in understanding less than nothing about yoga, never having practised it: he had only given it a superficial glance, and nobody would think of reproaching him on this account, had he not pontificated on the subject. Koestler can safely be left to his own devices: we would do better to listen to Swami

---

[1] Prana = energy, Sushumna Nadi = the channel of subtle energy corresponding in the material body to the spinal cord (see the passage at the end of this chapter by V. G. Rele).

Shivananda, the yogi-doctor, who tells us: 'Uḍḍīyāna Bandha is a blessing to mankind; it brings health, strength and long life to those who practise it. For abdominal exercises nothing can compete with Uḍḍīyāna and Nauli. They stand unique, unrivalled and unprecedented amongst all systems of physical exercises in the East and the West.'

THE MECHANICS OF UḌḌĪYĀNA

These are very simple, and easily understood after examination of the two photographs which follow.

After the lungs have been thoroughly emptied by a strong and forcible expiration, a mock inhalation is made in which the thorax is expanded, thus raising the diaphragm, which in turn drags the viscera up some way into the thoracic cage. Driven in by atmospheric pressure, the stomach hollows itself, vanishes and flattens. Seen in profile the abdomen has apparently disappeared.

METHOD

The following points are essential to success:

(a) The adept *must* be fasting.
(b) To allow the diaphragm to rise, the lungs *must* be emptied, and *must* remain empty throughout the exercise.
(c) The muscles of the abdominal wall *must be relaxed*, and must remain passive; if contracted, they would work against the action of the atmospheric pressure: *the abdominal muscles*, therefore, *are not brought into play at any point in the exercise*.
(d) The mock *thoracic inspiration* (i.e. the expansion of the thorax which does not result in the intake of air) is responsible for drawing the diaphragm up to its highest level.

POSITION

To achieve the correct position unerringly it is necessary at first to stoop down, so that the back is slightly rounded. Now rise up slowly, without altering the position of the trunk, that is to say without changing the inclination or the curvature of the back. When the legs are almost straight (in fact, the knees are bent as for ski-ing, the knee-cap being in a line with the toes), simply place the hands on the thighs, and you are in the correct position.

To relax the abdominal wall the arms must support the shoulders and keep the body firmly in place throughout the exercise[1] by pushing the elbows forwards, thus helping to make it all easier. Contract the neck and shoulders.

Position of the Feet

If you proceed as above, the feet will automatically be about 30 to 40 centimetres apart, and almost parallel one with another. When you are familiar with Uḍḍīyāna, you will be able to dispense with the first stooping position. The Bandha may also be practised while sitting in the Lotus posture.

BEGINNING THE EXERCISE

First Phase

Breathe out strongly, at the same time contracting the abdominal muscles, so as to empty the lungs *thoroughly*: the less residual air remaining in them the easier it will be to pull in the abdomen.

Second Phase

Without *allowing any air to enter* (a state known as apnoea), relax swiftly but completely the muscular wall of the abdomen which was contracted for the forcible expulsion of air from the lungs. Now expand the rib-cage, and imitate the movements of a deep thoracic inspiration. As soon as the ribs rise, the diaphragm moves up, and surprisingly, you will see the stomach moving inwards. Hold Uḍḍīyāna for a few seconds–five to begin with–and gradually increase the length of time.

Final Stage

At the end of Uḍḍīyāna allow the thoracic cage to resume its normal size, and the stomach to return to its normal position. Now, but only now, breathe in: the air will enter the lungs gently. If you allow air to enter during the Bandha, the depression in the thorax will cause it to rush violently into the lungs. In view of their very delicate structure, and the extreme fragility of the alveolar membrane, it is not advisable to induce this strain.

[1] Notice the position of the thumbs.

Uḍḍīyāna cannot succeed:

(a) If the lungs do not remain empty, and if you allow air to enter at the moment of drawing in the abdomen. *Remedy:* When you first start you may pinch the nostrils between the index finger and the thumb of the left hand, to make sure you are in a state of apnoea throughout the exercise.

(b) If the muscular structure of the abdominal wall remains in a state of contraction. In the starting position, lungs emptied, test the muscles in the stomach with your hand to make sure they are relaxed; otherwise Uḍḍīyāna will not be possible. *Remedy:* See next paragraph.

(c) If the expansion of the thoracic cage is insufficient. *Remedy:* lying on the back, try to bring in the stomach by expanding the rib-cage. It is easy to relax the stomach when lying down, and although it will retract to a much lesser extent, it will allow you to see how the movement is carried out.

AGNISARA DHAUTI

Uḍḍīyāna Bandha leads naturally on to Agnisara Dhauti. Agnisara Dhauti means literally 'purification through fire'. But you need have no fears–the fire refers merely to the fire of digestion. This Dhauti consists of a series of Uḍḍīyānas repeated without drawing breath: when the stomach is pulled in, allow it to return at once to its normal position, then pull it in again immediately, and so on until the need for air puts a stop to the exercise. Rest a little and then begin once more.

Proceed slowly at the start. Then step up the rhythm until the retraction takes place once a second in an uninterrupted series of fifty to sixty Uḍḍīyānas–or even more–without drawing breath.

There is no need to explain that, as in Uḍḍīyāna Bandha, the stomach must be empty.

The difficulty lies in carrying out these retractions while keeping the stomach totally relaxed. Agnisara Dhauti is unequalled for the manner in which it massages and churns the stomach region, thus making food easier to assimilate and speeding up the whole digestive process–the justification of the name, 'purification through [digestive] fire'.

215

Yogis make at least 500 retractions in this manner every day. which occupy, including the time taken for resting between postures, about five minutes. Some achieve as many as 1,000 or even 1,500 retractions. The Westerner may be content with a total of 100 or 150.

UDDĪYĀNA BANDHA: THE COMPLETE CLASSIC FORM

In this form of Uddīyāna Bandha, the oblique muscles must be made to stand out during retraction of the abdomen.

Concentrate upon contracting the sides, for it helps to isolate the oblique muscles. Do not be discouraged if success does not come immediately! There is so much to gain from even the simplified form, that you will be won over by an exercise which is the most beneficial of all.

CONTRA-INDICATIONS

These are all acute affections of the abdominal organs such as colitis, appendicitis and so on.

If the complaint were to be ignored the practise of Uddīyāna Bandha would cause pain. In this case you should stop, and consult your doctor. Prolapses on the other hand *are not* contra-indications and the exercise can be very helpful in these cases.

EFFECTS

Uddīyāna Bandha is a fundamental exercise which visibly affects the abdomen, thoracic cage and lungs. Its occult effects concern the awakening of Kundalini–the vital powers.

Effects upon the Abdominal Region

The viscera of all those leading a sedentary life, suffer from the superficial quality of the breathing, which deprives them of the rhythmic massage induced by the up-and-down movements of the diaphragm. The seated posture, moreover, induces stases of the blood in the viscera, to their detriment. A large quantity of blood is drawn off from the general circulation, thus sapping vitality. The digestion is upset, the work of the intestines slows down, resulting in a degree of constipation made all the more harmful by the conventional diet, which produces putrefaction in the intestines:

the toxins move through the intestinal wall, and succeed slowly but surely in poisoning the whole organism.

Uḍḍīyāna Bandha and Agnisara Dhauti correct this state of affairs by the deep massage and kneading of the viscera, and by speeding up of the abdominal circulation: every organ in the body benefits thereby. The whole of the digestive tract is stimulated –digestion is made easier, and dyspepsia banished. This statement would seem to contradict the essential feature in Uḍḍīyāna Bandha, which insists that the stomach must be empty before practise.

And so it must, but not necessarily the digestive tract! Once the stomach has done its work, the intestinal digestion continues for several hours.

The stomach benefits from Uḍḍīyāna, for its lower part is emptied of residual gastric juices. This is particularly the case with the prolapsed stomachs of modern 'good livers' which are more or less deformed and distended.

Uḍḍīyāna and Agnisara Dhauti influence the glands accessory to the digestive tract. The liver, situated beneath the diaphragm, is stimulated and decongested as well as the pancreas, where the Islets of Langerhans–which secrete insulin–are situated. The kidneys are toned up, diuretic action increases, the adrenal glands are stimulated, the genito-urinary tract is decongested, and renal prolapsus often cured.

The practice of Uḍḍīyāna decreases aerophagia; wind is evacuated, and the spleen stimulated and given increased activity.

Its Action on the Solar Plexus

·When dealing with the Bow posture, we spoke of the solar plexus as a nerve structure of the utmost importance. This abdominal brain helps in regulating every function of the abdominal region, and its action is widely spread throughout the nervous system. By the process of breath retention, Uḍḍīyāna acts on the pneumogastric nerve, and helps to regularize the balance of the involuntary nervous system.

Uḍḍīyāna Bandha stimulates the solar plexus by stretching the region and acts on the coeliac plexus as well.

Effects on the Thoracic Cavity

The abdominal region is not the only section of the body to benefit;

because Uḍḍīyāna Bandha causes a hollowing of the thoracic cage, so that the diaphragm, lungs and heart are all involved.

In so many civilized people the diaphragm is motionless and almost rigid. Yet it is designed to play a fundamental part in breathing its piston-like movements serving to massage the viscera and liven up the circulation of the blood. Uḍḍīyāna Bandha and Agnisara Dhauti restore the diaphragm to its normal mobility.

Uḍḍīyāna also works on the lungs, stimulating them as a whole, and restoring their elasticity, while apnoea in the emptied lungs serves to strengthen them. The heart which is carefully padded between the lungs, benefits from the massage induced through the repeated raising of the diaphragm on which it rests.

However, acknowledged sufferers from cardiac complaints must consult their doctor beforehand and refrain from these exercises.

CONCLUSION

Uḍḍīyāna Bandha and Agnisara Dhauti are a complete tonic treatment, and Swami Shivananda saw them justly as unequalled benefactors of humanity, without their equivalent in any other system of physical education.

Appendix

The following quotation from Vasant G. Rele,[1] an Indian doctor and yoga adept from Bombay, fully justifies the physiological and etymological claims made above for Uḍḍīyāna Bandha.

'The yogic asanas seek to maintain the body in perfect condition, by stimulating the circulation, the digestion, respiration, secretions and excretions . . . ! The literal meaning of Uḍḍīyāna Bandha is "restraint of the flying-up impulses". "Flying-up impulses" could only be afferent, and these afferent impulses within the body are generated by the sympathetic division of the autonomic nervous system, the larger part of which is located in the abdominal cavity. These impulses are catabolic or destructive in their activity, but they are curbed by the impulses from the other division of the same system, the parasympathetic – which are anabolic or preservative in their action. Thus between them these two divisions regulate the activity of the involuntary organs. There is restraint of the destructive activity

[1] *Yoga Asanas for Health and Vigour.*

of the parasympathetic, and in yogic parlance this is termed the awakening of the dormant Kundalini. The ancient sages have devised methods of rousing it by the indirect means of playing with the abdominal muscles . . .

'Excessive activity of the sympathetic nervous system inhibits peristaltic activity of the intestines and produces constipation. On the other hand, an excessive activity of the parasympathetic increases the movements of the intestines, and produces looseness of the bowels.

'In health, the balance of the rhythmic activity of the intestines is maintained by these two branches – sympathetic and parasympathetic – of the autonomic nervous system, acting unconsciously though antagonistically on each other. Over-activity of one part automatically stimulates the other part in order to counteract it.

'By the practice of Uḍḍīyāna Bandha the excessive activity of the sympathetic nervous system is controlled without exciting the parasympathetic, overstimulation of which would create a vicious circle. This disturbance of harmony between the two ultimately tends towards a loss of psychic balance, and may lead to mental derangement which may be manifested by anxiety, neurosis, suspicion, depression and restlessness; they are the outcome of emotional activities which are supposed to be under the control of the autonomic nervous system. The sudden retraction of the relaxed abdominal muscles, particularly the two recti (straight front muscles of the abdomen), against the spine after their preliminary contraction in the full expiratory effort in the practice of Uḍḍīyāna Bandha, drags the intestines upwards and downwards to their utmost limit. This stretches with them the sympathetic fibres curbing any tendency towards overactivity of the solar plexus – the brain of the sympathetic nervous system – without the stimulation of the parasympathetic . . .

'. . . The daily practice of these exercises not only massages and tones up the bowels to regain their normal rhythmic action, but in addition these exercises restore in a permanent and definite manner the unbalanced activity of the autonomic nervous system within the limits of normal physiological fluctuation.'

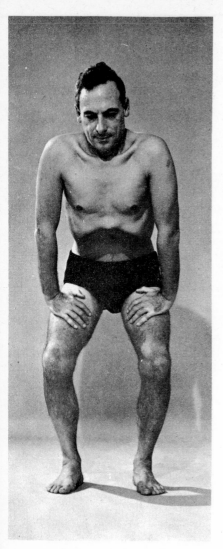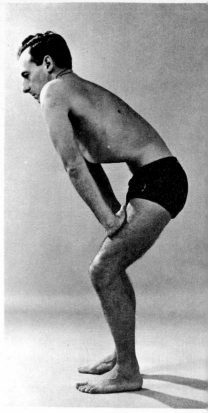

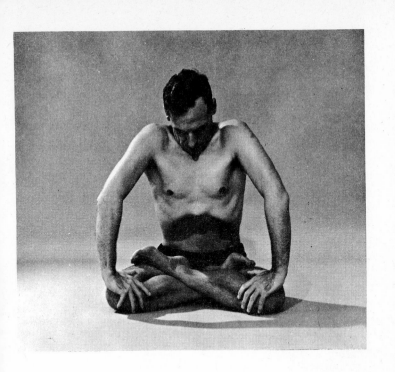

27. *Perfecting the Asanas*

An authentic Hindu hatha-yogi is an impressive sight in action. What strikes one most, apart from his absolute suppleness, is the harmony of his movements in the dynamic stage of the asanas. There is a total absence of hurried or jerky movements. The slow continuous progression is as peaceful and unrelenting as a river flowing through a plain. When, for instance, a yogi takes up the Plough posture, he raises his legs together from his recumbent position and carries his feet in a perfect arc to the floor behind his head.

He never for a moment loses control of the movement; he is clearly in perfect control of himself. The next posture is assumed in the same way, and he never ceases to breathe normally and easily. Expirations and inspirations succeed each other so harmoniously that he might be simply lying stretched out on the floor in a state of relaxation. His breath comes and goes like a wave over the sand. He is calm and serene: behind the movements of his body, one can sense the mental concentration, without the least tension, which commands this marvellous technique: the human body is here in perfect health, balanced, strong, obedient.

We should emulate him and try to carry out each movement of our yoga session in the same manner, so that we come to concentrate almost automatically, unaware of distractions. It is, in fact, impossible to be distracted if you are watching yourself strive for perfection, because so many different groups of muscles are successively coming into action and taking over from each other and any escape from this aspect of mental concentration becomes difficult.

Master the movement, controlling it throughout, keep your mind concentrated, calm and serene, and in this way you will discover true yoga, and experience renewed joy every day during your session of asanas.

In the period of immobilization, which is so clearly a central and essential feature, the yogi respects the definition of the asana as a position which is maintained (a) motionless, (b) for a long period, and (c) effortlessly.

Absolutely motionless, without twitching a muscle, the yogi holds the posture without the least discomfort. Only the coming and going of his breathing distinguishes him from a statue. Watch his face: it is as peaceful as a lake on a windless morning. Such perfection is not within the immediate reach of a beginner. but everyone should aim at it, and pursue it without pause; so that each day will bring a degree of further progress, of increased ease. comfort and added well-being and the maximum dividend of beneficial effects. You will soon reach the stage when you will wonder—so much have you become master of yourself and your forces—how you could ever have been satisfied with anything less.

The young and the less young may achieve this perfection of movement. each choosing postures according to his capability and ambition; he should bear in mind that yoga does not sanction acrobatics. Improve your technique. Aim at ease in movement and at immobility, and yoga will never become dull of tedious, but will inspire you to constant effort. The absolute mastery of mind over body is your aim and your reward. and both come from assiduous and persevering practice. Pay attention throughout to the relaxation of as many muscles as possible and employ the minimum of force in the dynamic stage; stay severely motionless in the static period without any superfluous tensing. Shīrsāsana is no exception, and your object is to find zero point, the point of perfect balance, in which the skeleton is stabilized in the posture, muscles relaxed, the body as still as a tower: you will feel that your body has become light, airborne.

28. *Sūryanamaskar*[1]: A Salutation to the Sun

You see how I write 'A' and not 'the' Salutation to the Sun: because there are several variants. I have chosen for this book the one which is taught in Swami Shivananda's ashram at Rishikesh, because it is accessible to everyone and easily learnt. A Salutation to the Sun is made up of twelve successive movements, repeated one after the other, which serve to bring the whole muscular structure into play, warming it up and 'conditioning' it for the asanas. It is an ideal exercise to get you moving, with more rapid movements than are customary in yoga: the speed of the performance will be indicated at a later stage.

A Salutation to the Sun however is a complete exercise, which may be practised outside the daily yoga session. By tradition yogis perform it only at dawn, before their asanas. Roman Catholics need not be alarmed! It is no pagan prayer and I have no intention of forcing anyone to carry out, unbeknownst to themselves, some Hindu ritual or other!

A Salutation to the Sun is a splendid exercise, and a yoga session without it is inconceivable. It prepares for the asanas and completes them, toning up the muscles, quickening and intensifying the respiration and cardiac rhythm, without inducing any fatigue or breathlessness. From the photographs it may seem that Sūryanamaskar is a very complex exercise, but do not be put off. In fact it is made up of just six movements, to be repeated in reverse. Start by learning the first four then work backwards, and take up positions 10, 11 and 12. Easy! Now learn movements 5 to 9. When you know it well you have only to place them in this sequence, and your Salutation will be complete.

But first of all listen to the Rajah of Aundh – a fervent advocate of the Salutation, who showed its effects on himself, his family, his entourage and even in the schools and workshops of his kingdom.

[1] Sūrya = Sun. Namaskar = salutation.

I must first warn you that this may all sound 'too good to be true'! And yet I have come more and more to appreciate the importance of Sūryanamaskar and its bountiful effects, here confirmed by the voice of the Rajah of Aundh:

Sūryanamaskar may be practised by anyone and everyone, singly or in a group, and at any time of the year, since it can be performed as well in a room as outside.

Sūryanamaskar takes only three to ten minutes a day.

Sūryanamaskar is not limited in its action to any one part of the body; it acts on the organism as a whole.

Sūryanamaskar costs nothing; there is no need of burdensome equipment. All you need is a space measuring two square metres.

Sūryanamaskar tones up the digestive system by the alternate stretching and compression of the abdominal region; it massages the viscera (the liver, stomach, spleen, intestines and kidneys), activates the digestion and gets rid of constipation and dyspepsia.

Sūryanamaskar strengthens the abdominal muscles and, by so doing, holds the organs in place. Blood stoppages in the abdominal organs are banished.

Sūryanamaskar synchronizes movement with breathing, thoroughly ventilates the lungs, oxygenates the blood and acts as a disintoxicant, because it gets rid of an enormous quantity of carbon dioxide and other toxic gases through the respiratory tracts.

Sūryanamaskar steps up cardiac activity and the flow of blood throughout the system, which is ideal for the health of the body. It combats hypertension and palpitations and warms the extremities.

Sūryanamaskar tones up the nervous system by successively stretching and bending the spinal column: it regulates the functions of the sympathetic and para-sympathetic systems and helps to promote sleep. The memory improves.

Sūryanamaskar allays worry and calms anxiety. The cells of the nerves recuperate more slowly than the others, but, with regular and assiduous practice, it will gradually restore their normal functions.

Sūryanamaskar stimulates and normalizes the activity of the endocrine glands—the thyroid in particular—through those movements which compress the neck.

Sūryanamaskar refreshes the skin, so that it takes on a gloss. A quantity of toxic products is evacuated through the skin and if the exercise is done correctly there is slight sweating and some moisture may appear. The Rajah of Aundh recommends that the exercise be continued until a profuse sweat is induced: in the Indian climate, a few minutes is enough but, under our skies, this is unnecessary. The skin is well irrigated, so that it reflects good health, and the complexion clears.

Sūryanamaskar improves the muscle structure throughout the body: neck, shoulders, arms, wrists, back, abdominal wall, as well as the thighs, calves and ankles, without inducing hardening hypertrophia in the muscles. Many forms of backache are easily and effectively held at bay because it strengthens the back.

Sūryanamaskar changes the appearance and deportment of the bust in women and girls. The bosom develops normally and becomes firm, regaining any lost elasticity, through stimulation of the glands and strengthening the pectoral muscles.

Sūryanamaskar controls activity in the uterus and ovaries, suppressing menstrual irregularity with its accompanying pain, and assists in childbirth.

Sūryanamaskar prevents loss of hair and reduces any tendency to greying.

Sūryanamaskar counterbalances the unfortunate effects of high-heeled or too tight shoes, belts, collars and other encumbering clothes. It prevents flat feet and strengthens the ankles.

Sūryanamaskar gets rid of any folds of fat, especially the surplus round the stomach, on the hips or thighs and on the neck and chin.

Sūryanamaskar reduces abnormal prominence of the Adam's apple: the neck in this exercise is bent forward, and the thyroid region is subjected to a rhythmic pressure.

Sūryanamaskar eliminates unpleasant smells produced by the body since it gets rid of toxins naturally through the skin, lungs, intestines and kidneys.

Sūryanamaskar increases immunity to disease by strengthening its potential breeding grounds.

Sūryanamaskar refines the proportions of the human body without causing hypertrophia of the muscles and by reducing excess fat.

Sūryanamaskar lends grace and ease to the movements and prepares the body for sport of all kinds.

Sūryanamaskar revives and maintains a spirit of youthfulness, an asset beyond price. It is wonderful to know that you are ready to face up to life and extract from it all the real joy it has to offer. To sum up,

226

Sūryanamaskar produces health and strength, and the efficiency and longevity which is the right of every human being.

The Rajah of Aundh concludes: If Sūryanamaskar is practised with integrity and perseverance it is not just a panacea. It rewards its adepts with superb health and vibrant energy, renewing youth in the elderly; through it, he says, his own life and the lives of the people dear to him have become a hymn of happiness. If you already know and practise the Salutation to the Sun, now is your opportunity to perform it more earnestly and more often than ever before.

If not, these pages will help you to an easy and agreeable apprenticeship.

Measure yourself round the thighs, waist, chest, neck and biceps. You will be convinced when in six months' time you come to re-measure and compare.

Work through each position separately for a few days, attempting the easiest ones first. Do not strive for instant perfection. One of Sūryanamaskar's main attractions is the constant potential of improvement you can bring to it.

Most descriptions of Sūryanamaskar fail to provide one essential piece of information: the rhythm of the movements. Too many people perform the Salutation to the Sun–in all good faith–as slowly as if it was an asana. This is to be regretted.

When you have a thorough knowledge of the Salutation you will be able to complete the twelve movements within twenty seconds.

Your first aim should be to do fifteen Sūryanamaskars in five minutes. After the first six months this is increased to forty in ten minutes. This is a useful average which may be divided into two sessions of, say, five minutes for a morning practice and a further five minutes in the evening before retiring. Women should not undertake the exercises during the first days of menstruation.

Expectant mothers may practise until the beginning of the fifth month: after the birth seek advice from the doctor and gradually reinstate your asanas.

Concentration is absolutely essential, and the conscious mind must play an active part in every movement. You must not think of anything else and you should avoid all distractions and interruptions. Maintain an uninterrupted rhythm throughout the succession of Salutations. The first ones, especially in the morning, may be slower and less developed, for the muscles will still be sluggish.

It is advisable to face the rising sun, or at least, to turn towards the east. Think of and concentrate on the sun, which invigorates the whole of life on this earth. Your entire energy, including that used in the Salutation, springs from its rays. At some given moment, every atom of your body was once part of the sun or of a star like it. Think of the cosmic force radiated by the sun. In this state of mind the content of the Salutation is heightened and infused with a spirit that transforms it from a seemingly ordinary muscular exercise into something which involves the whole personality.

If you know and are satisfied with a different variant of the Salutation continue with it. All are worthwhile exercises, but they should not be mixed together.

Among the variants, there is one which is infinitely more elaborate. In this version, the central passage, falling between the two inverted V-shape positions, is replaced by a plunging movement which is both very graceful and stimulating: but this calls for very sound wrists, arms and shoulders, as well as a supple back and a good muscular stomach.

It is essential to synchronize the breathing with the movements. Once again the difficulties only seem to be formidable, since synchronization is easy to achieve. If the adept co-ordinates his movements with his breathing, he will be able to perform his Salutations without running short of breath or energy.

Consult the diagrams which accompany the photographs over the next ten pages. This makes it easier to memorize the sequence of *breath-positions*. At first, while you are still unfamiliar with the movements, you need not bother with the instructions on breathing which will follow its natural course.

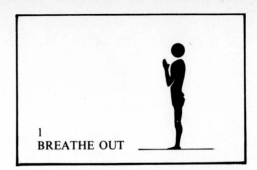

1
BREATHE OUT

A SALUTATION TO THE SUN

The correct twelve positions for A Salutation to the Sun are illustrated on the next ten pages. The breath rhythm for each stage is shown in diagram form at the top of each page. For six of these positions faulty postures are illustrated alongside the correct ones.

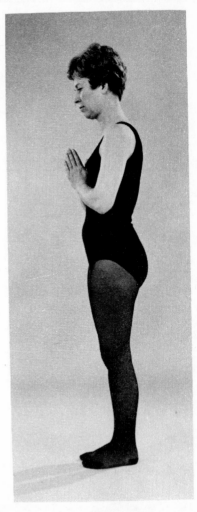

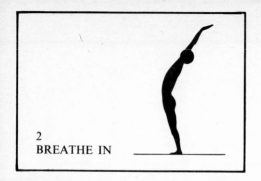

2
BREATHE IN

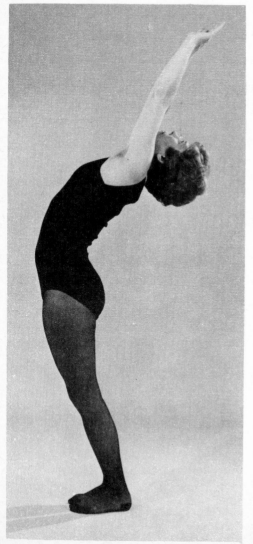

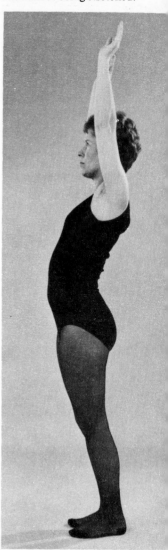

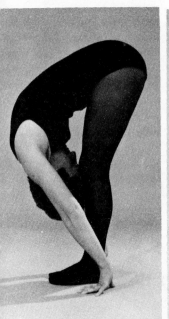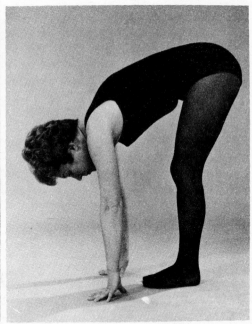

FAULT
The head has not been pushed towards the knees and therefore the curve is far less pronounced and its effects are correspondingly reduced. At this stage the thyroid is compressed by the pressure of the chin on the chest. In cases of imbalance of the thyroid, except in case of goitre—rare nowadays—and unless the doctor indicates otherwise, the asana will at the very least improve the situation.

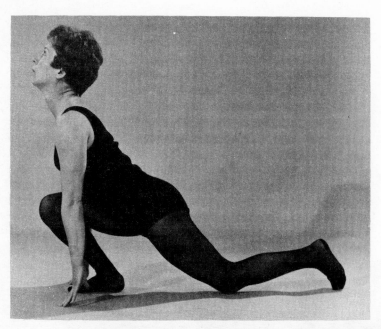

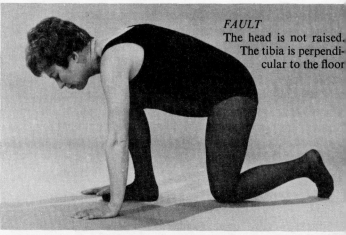

FAULT
The head is not raised.
The tibia is perpendi-
cular to the floor

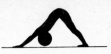
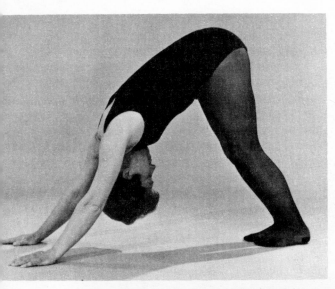

ULT
 heels do not
 ch the floor,
 body rises
 o the toes.
 body does
 form an
 erted V: the
 e has not been
 used on the
 al. The back
 ot stretched.
 e stomach
 ains
 ontracted.

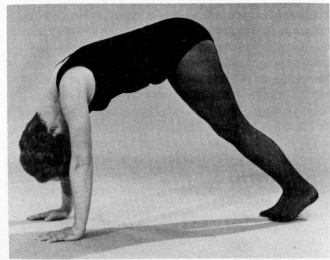

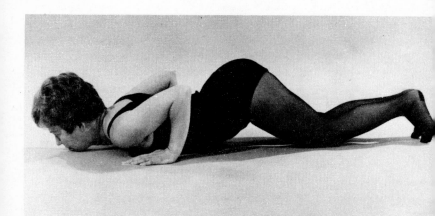
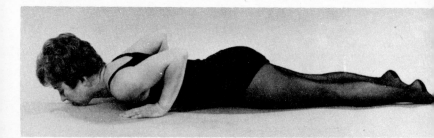

FAULT

Do not let the stomach lie flat on the floor, for the feet cannot be stretched out. The toes must remain on the floor.

Further, throughout the exercise, the hands should remain as though rivetted to the ground. The feet, once extended, remain in the same place on the floor, until they are brought back to their starting point at the end of the Salutation. To begin with, this will not be possible but you will be able to manage it in time.

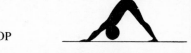

7
BREATHE IN

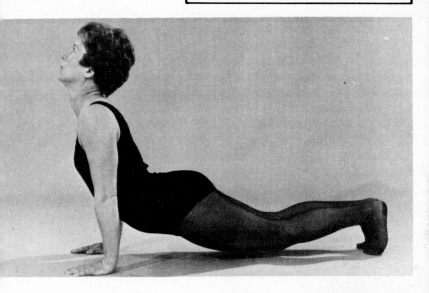

8
STOP

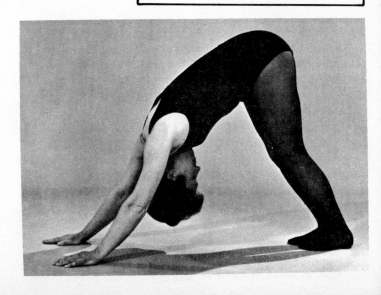

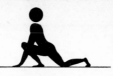

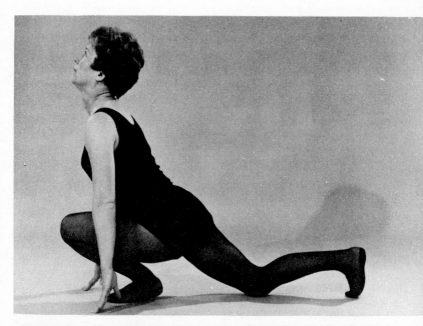

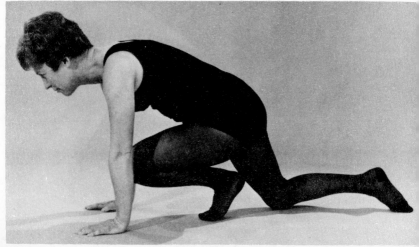

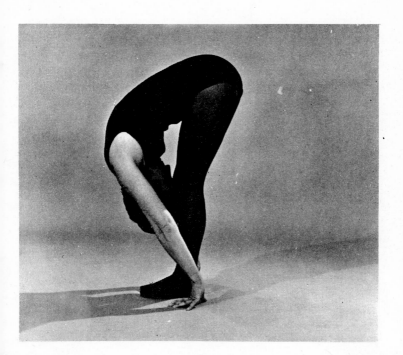

FAULT
Another mistake is illustrated here which follows from the two previous
ones: the feet are placed with their top surfaces instead of their toes
touching the floor. The leg is incorrectly bent. The left foot has not been
brought sufficiently close to the hands. At the outset, it is fairly hard to
bring back to the starting point. To ease this difficulty, settle the weight
of the body onto the opposite foot and hand; this allows the pelvis to tilt
slightly, thus easing the return of the foot.

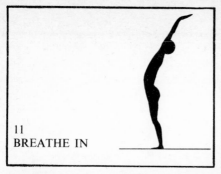

11
BREATHE IN

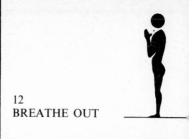

12
BREATHE OUT

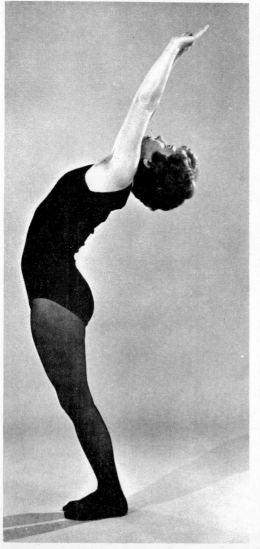

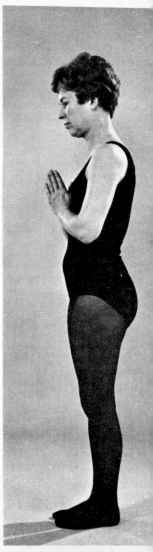

29. *We are What We Eat*

The Rishis of Ancient India laid down with infinite care the diet which keeps a yogi healthy and young; but the difference in climate and way of life, to say nothing of the food available, is such that in the West it is impossible to follow their precepts to the letter. The practice of yoga without attention to diet will never secure all the results which should be expected of it. Food is the material which builds the body and so we must establish dietary principles which are relevant to Western civilization. But this is not easy, because the various systems are surrounded by a web of argument and contradiction. The following pages will describe those fundamental principles on which almost everyone is agreed.

Let us first look at the main faults in our diet. Listen to the German specialist Dr W. Kollath:

'Except for illnesses resulting from accidental causes, poisoning (by lead, arsenic and so on), extremely virulent micro-organisms, and congenital malformations, most recognized illness stems directly or indirectly from improper feeding.'

In view of the conventional food eaten by the 'average' civilized being, it is really surprising that things are not worse. A growing number of people, although they are still in the minority, are aware of the situation. But it is a mistake to think that reforms in eating are merely concerned with actual food: it is, rather, a whole collection of feeding habits which has to be reviewed. I will list some of the more obvious ones.

WE SWALLOW FOOD:

   (i) too fast
  (ii) too hot – or too cold
 (iii) in too great a quantity
 (iv) adulterated, and
  (v) too rich, but at the same time impoverished.

The first three mistakes are the first to be remedied; if they are not, then most of the advantages of correct feeding are lost, while in avoiding them, if your diet is still open to discussion, at least some of the disadvantage will have been eliminated.

The essential factor lies in the assimilation of food and not in *what* you swallow.

Of course we know our food must be chewed thoroughly, because we were constantly reminded to do so at our primary schools, and this by a master who supervised the dining-room, where we bolted great slabs of bread and butter whole, and washed them down with brimming mugs of coffee.

Food which has not been properly chewed and so has missed the pre-digestive processes in the mouth, weighs on the stomach and intestines.

A yogi chews his food as patiently as a cow in order to extract all the taste; he will masticate until the mouthful liquifies, and then churn it round appreciably with his tongue – after the mucous lining of the nose, the main organ for the absorption of pranic energy. The well-known American dietician, Horace Fletcher, was not an inventor, but his work is worth studying, because he took his thinking farther than any of his predecessors. He is worthy of our respect because he puts his own theories into practice, which other 'system-makers' sometimes fail to do. Apart from the yogis, none before Fletcher had ever stressed the importance and the need for mastication, in such persuasive and irrefutable terms. Nor had anyone ever given such precise and practical instruction. If food is well chewed, it is half digested; when Fletcher chews it is three-quarters digested.

You must masticate, grind and churn every mouthful. Keep it in the mouth as long as you can, until it finds its way into the oesophagus. Do not count the number of your mastications! Allow the saliva to act on the food, while you concentrate entirely on the act of eating, on the variety of tastes which arise; you will come to find that food really does taste.

Digestion accounts for about sixty per cent of available nervous energy: by assisting in the very complicated work of the alimentary canal you free reserves of energy for other duties, whereas, if you do not chew your food enough, it becomes indigestible, causing digestive troubles and afflicting you with all the consequences of abnormal metabolism: dyspepsia, obesity or, in the opposite direction, excessive thinness.

Well-masticated, and so 'conditioned', the food reaches the stomach at an ideal temperature and you cut out the second and third mistakes, because those who eat too fast invariably eat too much. Any excess of even the best food is harmful. Because you will digest more easily you will feel better from your very first attempt to chew in the sensible manner.

One proof of the effectiveness of the method lies in evacuation: the stools are well-formed, soft, like damp clay and no longer smell bad: constipation is banished. You are familiar with its pernicious effects: how toxins produced by putrefactive bacteria pass into the blood, poisoning the whole system.

Fletcher also requires us to eat only when we are really hungry, while civilized man eats because it 'is time'. When real hunger sets in (there is all the difference between 'hunger' and 'appetite', which is only a desire to eat), the simplest dishes become delicious and the taste more subtle, while complicated food loses its attractions. You become an epicure in the real sense, while a glutton finds no real pleasure in even the most refined cooking.

Fletcher also says: 'Stop eating as soon as you feel satisfied—do not wait until you are replete!' He advises you to forget any worries and to argue after meals rather than before.

The change in your eating habits is a thankless task, which requires patience and perseverance. You must not delude yourself! It is very difficult to get rid of the deeply ingrained habit of eating fast. Many parents are guilty of pressing their children to eat quickly, even promising rewards to the one who finishes first, berating the last to finish with the threat of foregoing his pudding.

It is uncomfortable but essential to change the rhythm of chewing. Use the following method: put down your spoon, fork, or bread, place the hands in the lap and chew, with your eyes shut if possible, as an aid to concentration.

The first week is the worst, but you will soon find yourself unable to eat in any other manner.

Even liquids must be treated in the same way (soups, milk and so on), even water. Swami Satchidananda says: 'You must drink solids and masticate liquids.'

Nevertheless, you must not chew meat for too long as it then acquires a very bad taste: in any case there is no point in doing so, because meat is digested in the stomach by gastric juice and not by the ptyalin contained in the saliva, which is not the case with starchy foods.

Keep mastication for your cereal foods. Before ending this chapter I must confess that I myself eat too fast. Perhaps I should not have thrown a stone in my own glass house . . .

So you and I together will now agree to chew our next meal conscientiously and with determined energy. I hope you enjoy it!

30. *Carnivore or Vegetarian?*

The science of dietetics is not rewarding, because whatever the recommended regime, individual needs and circumstances prevent it from being universally acceptable.

If you ask a country dweller how to feed a horse, he will first enquire whether the animal is being worked or stabled. In the first case he will recommend a diet of oats; and in the second – of hay. Ask a racehorse owner the same question, and he will answer according to whether or not the horse is in training.

The same goes for human beings; but, in order to simplify a little we shall restrict our advice to 'sedentary civilized man' which, alas, we have nearly all become.

Whether to become vegetarian, or to go on eating meat? First of all, let me reassure you: it is not essential to cut out meat, just because you are practising yoga. In India yogis are vegetarian– lacto-cerealists to be precise: but this does not imply that the Westerner who practises for half an hour a day must likewise give up meat.

Let us leave our prejudices, however, while we consider the question and ask ourselves:

   (i) whether it is 'essential' to eat meat;
  (ii) if 'yes', then how much;
 (iii) if 'no', then why not, and also:
 (iv) what to replace it with.

It seems that amino-acids are essential, but these do not only occur in carcass meat. Let us not mince matters: the carnivore devours the entire corpse of animals which have often been dead for some time. What are the disadvantages of this?

1. Meat, that is to say muscle, is a food of little value, containing few vitamins and mineral salts. Its digestion makes demands on the

reserves of those vital substances which our food fails to provide in sufficient quantity, since commercialization is apparently bent on getting rid of them, by refining, by over-cooking at excessive temperatures and by 'industrial' treatment, all of which devitalize the food and remove essential minerals.

2. Meat contains excessive protein (animal, by definition) which upsets the metabolism and produces toxins (purine and the uric acids, the cause of rheumatism).

3. Muscle in animal carcasses contains all the organic waste of the slaughtered animal, in particular, a virulent poison known as xanthin.

4. Meat is a stimulant, which is why we like it. As with every other stimulant, the euphoria produced by it is followed by depression, so that in order to recapture the apparent state of 'well-being' it is necessary to resort to further stimulants (tea, coffee, tobacco) or to alcohol, the 'euphoric' *par excellence*. The consumption of meat, alcohol, tobacco and coffee is on an equal footing, because the use of one invokes the need of another.

5. In its natural form, meat is insipid and tasteless, only becoming palatable when cooked, grilled, and roasted. If raw, it is only eatable when heavily spiced and served with pickles or those sauces which in themselves contain substances detrimental to the organism.

No wild carnivorous animal would ever eat meat that had been salted and peppered.

6. It is not possible to live on meat without any vegetable supplement. The Eskimo and the Kirghiz races are not proper examples, since they are carnivorous only through absolute necessity. Moreover, not only do they eat muscle, but they also drink the blood and consume the entrails and other organs of animals. The Eskimos eat the contents of both stomach and intestines. Their average life-span lasts only twenty to twenty-six years: they die from arterio-sclerosis resulting from their diet of meat.

Carnivorous animals devour their prey in its entirety and derive their proteins, carbohydrates, fats, vitamins and mineral salts from the blood, liver, spleen, kidneys and bone-marrow rather than from the muscle. They even break up the bone, and invariably eat the cartilaginous tissue.

7. Meat, eggs and fish all have something in common; if they are left alone they putrefy rapidly. Milk does not putrefy but turns sour—a very different affair: cereals either grow mouldy or ferment, as do fruits and vegetables. The main disadvantage of

putrefaction has nothing to do with any effect on the taste but derives from the highly noxious toxins produced by the bacilli responsible for it.

The laboratory of the Public Health Service of the USA–which cannot be accused of prejudice–has carried out bacteriological research in order to establish the average number of bacilli causing putrefaction in a single gramme of the following:

Beefsteak	1,500,000 bacteria per gramme
Pork	33,000,000 bacteria per gramme
'Hamburger'	75,000,000 bacteria per gramme
Pork Liver	95,000,000 bacteria per gramme
Fish	110,000,000 bacteria per gramme
Eggs (a few days old)	200,000,000 on average

These putrefactive bacilli are our worst enemies. They invade the large intestine in their billions, and multiply there, changing the original bacterial flora which by right should contain a majority of fermentative bacilli, capable of dealing with cellulose tissue and playing no part in the manufacture of toxins. When putrefaction is set up in the large intestine, the enormous production of toxic products filters through the intestinal membrane, and slowly but surely poisons the system: these are the direct cause of innumerable organic changes by weakening the system and creating conditions favourable for the development of disease. When a 'hearty' eater leaves the lavatory the place is attended by an evil smell. Normal motions should be almost odourless.

The stubborn constipation which so many in our civilization have to endure often originates from this putrefaction, because the digestion of meat results in an insufficiency of faecal matter in the intestines, upsetting normal peristaltic action. The vegetarian who foregoes his regimen for a matter of days at once experiences this change in colour and smell, as well as a new difficulty in evacuating the bowels.

8. One more point for those willing to accept the facts: in eating meat you absorb animal vibrations which hinder your spiritual development.

If, in spite of everything, you must eat meat, eggs and fish, at least try to respect the following essential rules:

—Meat must be carefully apportioned; never eat more than 60 to 100 grammes (maximum!) a day.
—Avoid any kind of pork, beef is preferable.
—If you eat the meat well cooked, the number of putrefactive bacteria in the intestine is reduced. Beef tea, therefore, is sterile.
—Eggs and fish must be eaten *very fresh*.

Fresh fish is no problem with speedy transport and refrigeration, but eggs are a different matter, since those in the grocers' shops are rarely less than a week old, and often more like two or three. Even if they are hard-boiled for six minutes the bacilli are not killed.

If your stools smell badly, this is a sign that putrefaction inside the intestines is intense and you should counter it with the lactic germ (yoghurt) which checks the proliferation of the putrid bacilli and restores the acid balance in the intestines.

Our grandparents ate far less meat than we do today. Only thirty or forty years ago. meat appeared on the tables of country people once a day, in the shape of a piece of bacon, served with potatoes. The Sunday joint was 'an extra'.

One more piece of advice: eat meat as long as you feel you cannot do without it. The vegetarian must be one in spirit before he can become one at the table.

Do not be hurried! Convince yourself that it is possible not only to exist without meat, but that its absence will bring you immeasurable rewards in health. If you visit the cemetery of a Trappist Monastery, you will see that most of the monks (strictly vegetarian) lived to be almost a hundred and sometimes beyond. And the same is true of other vegetarian monastic orders. Cancer as well as arteriosclerosis is almost unknown among them, and so are coronary thrombosis and other types of degenerative illness—precisely the afflictions we most fear, and know least about, so that we are powerless to protect ourselves. But now the question arises: 'what do we substitute for meat?' The answer is: nothing! Your eating habits must be reviewed as a whole, and gradually, by stages, you must adapt yourself to the change-over. I must, however, make it clear once again that it is not essential to be vegetarian in order to practise yoga. What would happen to the butchers if everyone 'converted' themselves to vegetarianism?

In the first place no general conversion of this sort could take place overnight; we can hardly hope that the trade would emulate one of my oldest friends, who practised yoga and ran a butcher's shop; he used to advise his astonished customers to give up meat because it was unhealthy, and so on. He ended by closing his shop and opening a vegetarian restaurant!

31. *Adapting your Diet*

You can improve your diet without revolutionising your eating habits. as long as you substitute alternatives gradually; the diet. though still imperfect, will be a great improvement upon conventional feeding.

Here are some easy alternatives:

WHOLEMEAL RATHER THAN WHITE BREAD

White bread under its golden crust looks soft and delicious – but, alas, it is solid starch and nothing more. Replace it with good quality bread made out of wholemeal flour.

It may remind you of wartime shortages and it looks rather less attractive than the white kind; but it is a food of the highest nutritional value and the only one worthy of the name 'bread'.

There are many delicious brands, so choose one from the many different firms which bake it. The flour should contain the germ of the wheat. You will soon come to prefer it, and you will look upon white bread as being as tasteless as cotton wool. You will come to eat wholemeal bread by itself, without needing jam or anything else. Bread worthy of the name is enough in itself.

It requires prolonged chewing which makes it easy to digest by even the most delicate stomach. and its delicious taste is not properly brought out until it has been masticated for some time.

CUT OUT REFINED WHITE SUGAR

Commercialized white sugar is a purely chemical production, and the less you eat of it the better. Since our bodies manufacture their own sugar from cereals, they need no extra supply. Humanity would have become extinct by now had sugar been really essential, since it has only come into use quite recently. Refined white sugar extracted from beet dates from the English blockade of Europe under Napoleon. Ever since, production and, therefore, consumption has risen to the astonishing heights reached today.

Your way of life need not be thrown to the winds, for you can replace the ordinary white sugar with that made from unrefined cane sugar in the form of moist brown sugar, such as Demerara.

In the days of Louis XIV, sugar was such a rare commodity that the Sun King locked away precious cane-sugar brought back from 'the islands'. Some decades later it could be bought from the chemists or apothecaries, as they were known then.

DOWN WITH REFINED SALT. UP WITH SEA-SALT!

Ordinary white salt is also made from chemicals. Sodium Chloride— to use its correct name—has been refined and has therefore lost its oligo and other vitally important elements. Admittedly it stays dry in damp weather and pours easily from the salt-cellar without blocking the holes: and it is reassuringly white . . .

What does that matter? Replace it with sea-salt. In soup, or other dishes, nobody will notice the difference but your body will know all about it. Blood plasma, remember, is sea-water in diluted form!

ANTI-CHOLESTEROL-FORMING FATS PREFERRED

Civilized man eats too much and too richly. When it comes to fats, the quality is all-important. Reduce the supply of lipoids in general, but be severe in the avoidance of hydrogenated fats, rich in saturated fatty acids: this includes all solidified fats (ordinary margarines, cocoa butter, etc.) and animal fats! Use oil from the first cold pressing of soya, the germ of wheat or maize, which lowers the level of cholesterol in the blood, and prevents arterio-sclerosis (hardening of the arteries). All oil which has been manufactured into solid form has lost its entire content of non-saturated fatty acids, which are closely related to vitamins.

The only acceptable margarine is one based on sunflower—non-hydrogenated. Compared with butter it looks anaemic and unappetizing, but no one could wish it 'coloured' simply to please the eye.

Reduce your intake of fats therefore and use only anti-cholesterol-forming oils, and you will be doing your heart and arteries a power of good.

MORE RICE, LESS POTATO

The humble potato has its own indisputable qualities—being rich in mineral salts and vitamin (C), and in view of the over-acid quality of the food eaten by civilized man, it has the most useful basifying qualities. But this is not enough to afford it the place of honour in our diet. It is best to eat it only on occasions, perhaps once or twice a week, and to replace it otherwise with rice—whole rice, of course, and not the ordinary glazed variety. None of the gourmets of your acquaintance will complain, since rice can be prepared in a thousand ways, each more delicious than the last. It is a food of very high dietetic value and should figure largely in your diet. It should become the foundation of your main meal.

Potatoes should be cooked in their skins which should be removed immediately after cooking: if you fail to do this, you are throwing their soluble mineral salts down the sink.

EAT FRUITS IN SEASON

The fruits of our soil are balanced biologically with ourselves. Eat them in their season when they have ripened naturally on the tree. Do not refuse all exotic fruit on principle, but do cut down on it. Oranges which have ripened in the sun rather than in the hold of a ship are far better. Bananas are best left out altogether, for they have invariably been ripened in this way. Eat nuts as well—almonds, hazel-nuts and roast chestnuts in season.

AVOID TINNED FOODS

Fresh country vegetables, grown if possible without the use of chemical fertilizers, are better than any tinned food, which is guaranteed to keep for an indefinite period. But—this is only achieved after up to as many as seven successive cooking processes. What possible value remains in these products? Of course it is impossible to avoid them altogether in the civilized world, but do cut them out as far as you can.

32. *The Kollath Breakfast*

Our planet shelters 700,000 different species of living things, but only man and the animals he has domesticated feed on cooked foods. Natural food should be raw, but alas, our stomachs and intestines are unable to cope with it – especially in cereal form; for we are not like the grain-eating birds which pre-digest food in the crop.

Professor Werner Kollath, who is a dietician as well as a doctor of medicine, has found a way to make wheat digestible without cooking it. This 'Kollath breakfast', is not to be confused with Bircher-Muesli which is based on fruit (grated apple, especially), condensed milk, lemon juice and a small quantity of oat flakes – and designed to increase the consumption of fruit with cereals as only a secondary ingredient.

The Kollath breakfast is intended to make wheat easily digestible without cooking; the fruit is added to improve the taste and to complete the food value.

HOW TO PREPARE THE 'KOLLATH BREAKFAST'

The basic recipe is as follows: ingredients for one person are: 20 to 40 grammes (2 to 3 tablespoons) of fresh whole wheat flour. 3 to 5 spoonfuls of water, 1 to 2 spoonfuls of lemon juice: 15 grammes of dried fruit finely chopped, 100 grammes of apples – grated just before serving – or of any other fresh fruit in season – 1 tablespoon of ground almonds or hazel-nuts to scatter over the whole.

In the evening: Place 30 to 40 grammes of fresh wheat-flour into a bowl (your electric coffee-mill will grind wheat grains into flour in a few seconds). Add 3 to 5 spoonfuls of water, but *never* milk.

Stir, then leave it at room temperature ($+20°C$) until the next morning. The cereal will go on swelling through the night, and by morning it will have become a firm paste, and chemical changes will have taken place through fermentation – a process responsible for the value as well as the digestibility of the Kollath breakfast.

In another vessel soak 15 grammes of dried fruit.(figs, raisins or dates–finely chopped).

Next Morning: Mix the contents of both vessels using the water in which the dried fruit was soaked, and adding 1 to 2 spoonfuls of fresh lemon juice, together with 100 grammes of grated apples or pears, or any other fruit in season: crushed cherries, strawberries, plums, peaches, etc.

Dust the mixture with the crushed almonds or hazel-nuts.

You can vary the mixture according to taste, adding fresh cream, almond paste, or hazel-nut spread, or alternatively a teaspoonful of honey. Each person should be given 4 to 6 tablespoons of the mixture. The apple must be grated just before serving so as to avoid oxidation (always use a stainless steel grater), because the pulp must remain white. The meal should be juicy but not liquid.

If you are still hungry *afterwards* you may eat a little wholemeal bread, with white cheese made from skimmed milk.

Regular use of Kollath's breakfast will result in these effects:

(a) A feeling of satisfaction for at least the next four hours. No false hunger during the morning–no bloated sensation in the stomach;

(b) The weight will adjust itself. Those who wish to slim will not feel hungry before luncheon and therefore will not require so large a meal. Those, on the other hand, who wish to put on weight will find their digestion improving, and with this there will be an increase of weight. It seems paradoxical, but is in fact quite logical.

(c) Constipation, a factor in auto-intoxication is banished. Because this breakfast is a disintoxicant, any signs of tiredness and exhaustion which point to the accumulation of toxins, rather than to real fatigue, will disappear.

(d) Physical and intellectual efficiency increases;

(e) There is a feeling of general well-being which comes from improved biological balance.

(f) Inner happiness and satisfaction, banishing all desire for stimulants such as coffee, tobacco or alcohol.

(g) The powers of concentration increase, because the digestive system is not encumbered with a heavy meal. Remember that the digestion accounts for 70 per cent of available nervous energy.

(h) Resistance to stress improves.

(i) So does the composition of the blood. The multiplication of the cells of the skin resulting from better irrigation of the sub-cutaneous tissues makes the complexion rosy and banishes eczema, boils and dry skin.

(j) The hair becomes supple and alive. Dr Kollath has even cited cases where regular use of this breakfast formula has put a stop to greying hair and allowed the normal colour to return.

(k) The nails become shiny, and lose their brittleness.

(l) The teeth improve. Dr Kollath can cite instances where paradentosis, for which so far no cure has yet been found, has not only been arrested, but has retrogressed. Teeth which had become loose have tightened in their sockets, according to the evidence of Dr H. Netter.

(m) The skeletal structure is strengthened, so that fractures become less common, and, if an accident occurs, the bones knit more quickly.

Cereals and fruit taste well together in the Kollath breakfast. The odour of the fresh-ground flour is blended with the fragrance of the fruit. Carefully prepared, the breakfast becomes a delicacy varied in its composition by the use of seasonal fruits. The fruit adds its juicy freshness to the cereal, and by stimulating the salivary glands, assists, from the moment it enters the mouth, in preparing the alimentary bolus, so that the food is better assimilated and with the least expenditure of energy. The vitamins of the B complex found in fresh flour are added to the vitamin content of the fruit. Organic acids in fresh fruit are neutralized by the carbohydrates in the cereal. Preparation is easy, and uncomplicated, since there is no morning cooking required at a time when there is often hardly a minute to spare.

Try it faithfully for a few weeks and see the results!

33. *Eat Wheat*

Every human race has built itself up on a cereal food. For the Asians, rice, in the West, wheat or barley. Whole cereal is the best staple diet of all, and the Kollath breakfast is a complete ration in itself. But here is another way to prepare wheat: one of the oldest known, even older than baking. This is boiled wheat or porridge.

Even at this moment three-quarters of humanity still lives on a diet of boiled bread grain, cooked in fresh water or milk. We must therefore call upon man's oldest friend – fire. But does heat destroy living properties in the wheat? In this case that risk is minimal, because the temperature must be raised above 160°C to produce any important changes, and in boiling water the temperature cannot by definition exceed 100°C which is below the critical threshold.

It is essential to use fresh flour, milled just before use – there should be no difficulty in this because of the electric coffee-mill, which most households possess. The flour should be used immediately, otherwise the most precious and least stable content will soon oxidize and be lost.

Proceed as follows:

Grind a small quantity of wheat. Dilute a tablespoonful of unrefined cane sugar in a bowl of hot water. Add a tablespoon of sunflower oil or corn, soya or other good quality oil from the first cold pressing. Use no salt. Mix well with a fork and beat the liquid. Now pour the flour and contents of the bowl into a fireproof dish. The proportion of water should be such that the mixture is too thin at the beginning, for it thickens as it cooks.

Bring slowly to the boil, which will thicken the mixture, and then cook for ten minutes at least, stirring all the time, add water (or milk if you prefer) if the mixture thickens too much, or threatens to stick – it should be smooth and creamy. After cooking add raisins, almonds, ground hazel-nuts, grated coconut or apple, etc. You can vary the taste indefinitely.

If you wish, you may add cane-sugar or honey.

This delicious and nutritive dish will give you the feeling of having eaten 'well', although the quantity of wheat in the mixture is minimal.

Children adore this porridge, preferring it to advertised commercial products with a base of cocoa, white flour and sugar.

It is a delicious way to add whole cereal to your diet and this dish adjusts any weight problem: the over-thin person will gain and the overweight will thin down.

Try it, enjoy your meals, and you will soon be telling everyone how good it is.

Note: This porridge may be prepared without using oil. A number of other cereals such as rye, barley or rice, may be prepared in the same way, or alternatively the cereals may be mixed together: for example 80 per cent of wheat with 20 per cent of buckwheat, thus increasing the range of flavours still further. Eat this porridge and the Kollath breakfast on alternate occasions: the latter preferably for breakfast, with porridge at the evening meal. It may be given to all young children, provided care is taken to grind it very finely, and to cook it for a longer period (20 minutes), so as to make it more soluble and facilitate its digestion.

This whole and balanced food suits everyone including even those with the most delicate stomachs. Masticate it carefully, even though it is almost liquid.

34. *And Finally . . .*

This book, which seems opposed to the principle that yoga should only be taught to the initiated—that is to say through the direct teaching of Master to disciple—cannot hope to deal exhaustively with the subject in a few hundred pages.

What it can do is to allow the pupil, safely and in private, to assimilate the right techniques of yogic breathing and relaxation, as well as the principal asanas, which bring health, vitality and *joie de vivre*.

And are the Masters outmoded, outmatched or redundant? By no means. The adage of yoga: 'When the disciple is ready the Master appears', is as true today as it was four thousand years ago.

The adept is right to prepare himself through personal study for the blessing of *his* Master's message for which this book prepares the way. Are teachers of yoga redundant? The author, who teaches in his own Institute in Brussels, does not think so. Far from it—he believes that this work reinforces the value of the true teacher, who contributes infinitely more by guiding his disciples along the complete way of yoga—far beyond the asanas.

Let us once again remember the words of Swami Shivananda: 'An ounce of practice is worth several tons of theory.'